ALSO BY LYNDA HUEY

The Waterpower Workout
(R. R. KNUDSON)
A Running Start: An Athlete, A Woman

The Complete Waterpower Workout Book

The Complete Waterpower Workout Book

*Programs for Fitness,
Injury Prevention, and Healing*

**Lynda Huey
Robert Forster, P.T.**

Photographs by Pete Romano

Random House
NEW YORK

The Waterpower Workout is a registered service mark of Huey's Athletic Network.
For permission to teach The Waterpower Workout program in the sequence
contained in chapters 2 and 3, please contact Huey's Athletic Network on (310)
829-5622 between the hours of 9 a.m. and 5 p.m. (Pacific time) Monday through
Friday.

Library of Congress Cataloging-in-Publication Data

Huey, Lynda.
   The complete waterpower workout book : programs for fitness, injury
  prevention, and healing / by Lynda Huey and Robert Forster, PT ;
  photographs by Pete Romano.—1st ed.
      p.   cm.
  Published simultaneously in Canada.
  Includes index.
  ISBN 0-679-74554-8
   1. Aquatic exercises. 2. Aquatic exercises—Therapeutic use.
 I. Forster, Robert, PT. II. Title.
 GV838.53.E94H84   1993
 613.7'16—dc20   92-34286

Book design by Richard Oriolo

Manufactured in the United States of America

4 6 8 9 7 5 3

Preface
by Lynda Huey

When *The Waterpower Workout* was first published in 1986 by New American Library, it was the most comprehensive book of the very few in the new water-training field. It presented the most current information then available and drew heavily on my own experience and imagination.

As I designed my Waterpower Workout programs, I used my awareness of human movement from teaching swimming and my years of coaching basketball, volleyball, field hockey, and track and field. I used insights I had gained from my own struggles to keep my fitness while injured with ankle sprains, Achilles tendinitis, and hamstring strains. I used sports medicine knowledge from journals and applied it to water rehabilitation programs I created at the International Sportsmedicine Institute in Los Angeles. I studied basic sport-specific movements, broke them down into smaller component parts, then created water exercises aimed at developing strength in the major muscles used in sports. Finally, I tried to imagine the future: what water-training equipment would be developed to make my programs even more exciting and helpful.

The discovery of my Waterpower program by high-profile athletes (Florence Griffith Joyner, Wilt Chamberlain, Jackie Joyner-Kersee, John Lloyd, and Mike Powell, among others) took water exercising from where it had languished in obscurity and placed it in the forefront of athletic training programs. Here was an activity that offered an injury-free environment for high-powered training—and athletes loved it. They spread the word about water in newspaper interviews and on television, and among themselves. Soon I had hundreds of people calling me for information about water training. Among these people were coaches and their injured athletes, dancers, pregnant women, marathoners, arthritis patients, aerobics instructors, triathletes, basketball players, yoga devotes, mountain bikers, multiple sclerosis patients, injured step-aerobics enthusiasts, soccer players, actors and actresses needing to look good on camera, gymnasts, amputees, men and women seeking fitness in a user-friendly exercise environment, power walkers, wrestlers, football players, people who had recently had surgery, people who were trying to avoid surgery, and people wanting to get in shape prior to surgery. Water was the great equalizer. I could give dozens of these people workouts, all at the same time in the same pool. Then once they learned my programs, they could enter any pool or private water tank or calm river, lake, or ocean and emerge after the workout refreshed, trained, and on their way to healing.

Since my last book, I feel as though I've had a lifetime of experience. I've taught Waterpower and Deep Waterpower Workout classes at UCLA. While there I've worked with coach Bobby Kersee, cross-training his Olympic athletes—Andre Phillips, Gail Devers, Valerie Brisco, and Al Joyner among them. During the 1988 Olympic Games I gave Waterpower Workouts at the Seoul Hilton indoor pool. Then I found myself pulled into postoperative water therapy in California, Florida, New York, Australia, and elsewhere. I helped rehabilitate an urban cowboy with two total knee replacements, a television executive recovering from back surgery, and a ballet dancer who had total hip replacement surgery. Soon these patients were explaining water's benefits to their own doctors, and I was getting referrals from orthopedic surgeons. I worked with professional tennis player John Lloyd, showing him the benefits of water in helping the body gain coordination and symmetry in a unilateral (one-sided) sport. I helped rehab a major knee reconstruction for recreational tennis player Wilt Chamberlain, the former NBA great, then designed another program for his arthritic hip.

As I traveled and lectured, I spread my experience to other sports professionals. Herm Schneider, trainer for the Chicago White Sox, read about my work with Olympic sprinters and asked me to help him design a water speed-training program for the recovering Bo Jackson. Several months later, dancer and singer Paula Abdul asked me to help her recover from knee surgery in time to resume her 1992 world tour. Then actress Cybill Shepherd asked me to design a karate-specific Waterpower Workout for her prior to the filming of the TV movie *Stormy Weathers*. At the 1992 Olympic Track and Field Trials, coach Randy Huntington and his long jumper Mike Powell joined with me to help teach the international media about using Waterpower Warm-Downs after every track workout.

Seven years ago there was no water-training equipment on the market except for basic flotation belts and tethers. Today, much of the water-fitness equipment I dreamed of is a reality. These and other water products pictured here in *The Complete Waterpower Workout Book* will be explained, and their uses demonstrated.

Many clients have added covers to their pools so they can heat them and exercise in them year round. In order not to miss a workout in cold weather, many of us use Wet

Wraps, shortie wet suits, or full-length wet suits. The only negative trend in water exercise that I have observed over the past ten years is the increase in the building of "shallow water only" pools. When a swimming pool does not have deep water (over seven feet), half of the programs contained in this book cannot be performed and therefore half the benefits cannot be obtained. Keep that in mind if you are considering building a pool, or if you are searching for a public pool for your workouts.

The first half of the book, "Waterpower," teaches my basic shallow and deep-water programs and provides additional programs for athletes and dancers. The second half of the book is "Water Healing." Because many people come to water for the first time during the crisis of an injury, I've added six chapters on rehabilitation. To gain additional knowledge for these chapters, I asked physical therapist Robert Forster to coauthor this book with me and orthopedic surgeon Dan Silver to contribute his expertise. Robert and I have worked side by side with many of the same athletes, and we both bring a cautious, yet aggressive approach to their rehabilitation. Over the years he has used Waterpower as an integral part of his physical therapy programs, sending both elite and recreational athletes to the pool for rehabilitation or cross training. His training and experience provided a solid scientific foundation to back up my concepts. Dr. Silver has pioneered many arthroscopic surgery techniques in the past twenty years and is "the dance doctor of L.A." He collaborated on Chapter 11, Postsurgical Water Healing. The three of us feel confident that you will find what you need to move through your rehabilitation all the way back to your own personal gold medal, whatever that may be. For some of you, the gold actually means a win at the Olympic Games. For most of you, gold probably means the return to full functioning in your homes, careers, and recreational sports.

In 1986, a half million Americans were regular participants of "vertical" water exercise, which is a record-keeping term for aquatic exercisers who are not lap swimmers. Today their numbers have jumped to 6 million! This explosive growth proves what I've been saying in clinics and interviews for the past seven years: In the 1960s it was tennis: in the seventies, the running craze began; in the eighties, it was aerobics.

Now, water is the way of the nineties.

Santa Monica, 1992

Preface

ix

Preface

by Robert Forster, P.T.

For a clinical health-care practitioner there is nothing more rewarding than providing patients with exercise regimes, or knowledge about their injuries, that they will use in their daily lives long after treatment is completed. Sometimes they even pass what's been taught on to their friends. In this way one's work is not limited to current patients but extends to a much wider audience.

And so it gives me great pleasure to share in this book the knowledge I have gained from thirteen years of clinical practice as a physical therapist and from years of competitive and recreational sports experience as an athlete.

I first worked with water therapy in high school while rehabilitating my own sports injuries. Later while working at my first physical therapy position with patients suffering from knee, hip, and back problems, I learned more about the great benefits of exercising in water. Water offered freedom of movement and security to injured patients as no other exercise medium could. I knew water therapy and exercise had a very promising future.

The beginning of my career in physical therapy and rehabilitation coincided with the start of the modern fitness movement of the 1970s. People all over the country joined the running craze believing that it would protect them against disease, help them lose weight, and feel better, and because it was fun.

This fitness movement found the medical community unable to provide rational care for an active general public. Certainly there were doctors and therapists who were involved with the care of professional and elite athletes but the family doctor and general physical therapist were poorly trained to deal with a case of shin splints or a sore knee suffered by an accountant or lawyer caught up in a new life-style of fitness.

My colleagues and I were among the first to be trained in school to deal with these exercise ailments in the general public. At the State University of New York at Stony Brook we were taught that as physical therapists we were in the perfect position not only to evaluate and treat sports injuries but also to help critique and design fitness and sports-training programs. Since we witness first hand how the body typically breaks down and are trained to help fix it, who can better act as a conduit of information from the worlds of medicine and research to the athletes, coaches, and fitness instructors who desperately need guidance in establishing training programs that maximize fitness and performance while minimizing injury? We were made to feel that along with our education came a responsibility in preventative medicine, to help steer the public along its journey to health and well-being. Conversely we borrowed from the research in fitness and exercise and applied it to the construction of rehabilitation programs. From the start of my professional career I incorporated ideas and philosophies of fitness into each and every treatment program carried out at my Santa Monica, California, physical therapy clinic. Every patient becomes an athlete, at least while rehabilitating at our center. And those who aren't athletes before, commonly continue with the exercise and fitness programs we devise as part of their rehabilitation after they return to full health.

Exercise is the mainstay of our rehabilitation programs because the body is a mechanical device which requires mechanical treatment (exercise) to mend what ails it. Furthermore, to keep fit during rehabilitation is to satisfy the first tenet of sports medicine. These ideas provide the basic premise of this book. Exercising in water has proved to be the most exciting new development in both sports medicine and fitness. Water provides a perfect medium for rehabilitation exercises and is a forgiving environment for fitness training for persons of all ages and physical condition.

Working with coach Bob Kersee and his Olympic athletes I have discovered anew the power of water therapy. In the 1980s while rehabilitating injured athletes such as Valerie Brisco and Al Joyner I saw them struggle using the bicycle or with other cross-training activities until their recovery had progressed enough to allow for a return to running. When Lynda Huey developed her water exercise programs we found injured athletes could maintain fitness running in the pool with little chance of aggravating their injuries. Water exercise not only kept them fit but complemented the physical therapy they received in the clinic. In 1984 when Jackie Joyner-Kersee strained her hamstring just two weeks prior to the Olympic Games I began aggressive physical therapy and used water training to keep her running and jumping—to the heptathalon silver medal. Many similar success stories have followed and water therapy has become a permanent adjunct to my rehabilitation programs.

When Lynda Huey approached me with the idea of writing a comprehensive water-exercise and rehabilitation book I saw the opportunity to match her innovative water-exercise programs with the latest in scientific training principles.

Whether you use water training as your sole fitness activity or for cross-training purposes the first half of the book will teach you to construct a year-round training program. You will learn the various aspects of physical fitness and how to vary workouts to achieve each one while avoiding overtraining and injury. You will learn how to warm up, work out, and warm down like today's Olympians.

The second half of the book, "Water Healing," will teach you the principles of injury, healing, and rehabilitation that I have come to rely on when designing physical therapy programs for Olympic and professional athletes. The specific rehabilitation exercises found here when performed in the context of the Water Healing Workout provide therapeutic benefits for your injury while you maintain your fitness.

In the midst of today's health insurance crisis more and more Americans are finding themselves responsible for more of their own health care, especially when physical injuries strike. This book can help. After an injury occurs the first step is to obtain an accurate diagnosis from a doctor; then, perhaps more importantly, you should receive an evaluation from a physical therapist to establish the exact amount of dysfunction associated with your injury. The physical therapist will also identify factors such as tight or weak muscles that may have contributed to the cause of your injury. With this information you can set out to rehabilitate your injury while you maintain or even improve your overall fitness using The Waterpower and Water Healing Workouts.

It is my hope that this book will also serve as a manual for water therapists, coaches, athletes, and fitness instructors turning to water for all its wonderful benefits in cross-training and fitness development. Good luck and have fun!

Santa Monica, 1992

A c k n o w l e d g m e n t s

The following people contributed to the success of this book:

For Lynda Huey, Alexis Estwick, Patti Ballard, Janvie Cason, and Nirvana Gayle kept the high watch in the spritual realm while Tim Hoy, Wilt Chamberlain, Margie Mulligan, Glenn and Bob Huey supplied personal insight and reassurance.

For Bob Forster, special appreciation to his parents: Robert, Sr., for instilling the courage to chase dreams, and Madeline for teaching compassion.

Dr. Dan Silver collaborated on Chapter 11, Postsurgical Water Healing, and let us shoot the cover photo in his pool.

Pete Romano was extremely generous with his talents and his time in shooting the interior photos of the book. Matt Brown and Jay Herron were quick on their feet as his photo assistants. Joel Lipton brought his artistic eye to the cover photos. Anne Kresl shot Lynda Huey's head shot and Kathy Hostak was the makeup artist. John Livzey shot the two photos of Jackie Joyner-Kersee. Jill Freed shot several photos at UCLA.

Leroy Perry, Jr., D.C., invited Lynda Huey to help him create pioneering water exercise and water therapy programs at his International Sportsmedicine Institute in 1983, and there the work contained in this book began. Dr. Perry developed the floating traction shown in Photo A, page 263, and assisted-swimming exercises 17–21 in Chapter 9.

Clifton Mereday, Ph.D., P.T., chairman of the Physical Therapy School of the State University of New York at Stony Brook, challenged his student Robert Forster not only to create successful rehabilitation programs but also analyze and design health and fitness programs for safety and effectiveness.

Anne Martini and Judith Sperling at UCLA both believed in The Waterpower and Deep Waterpower Workouts and gave valuable pool space for programs that aided students, faculty, and many top athletes. UCLA allowed us to shoot several photos there.

Rosalynn Krissman warmly invited us to shoot the majority of the book's photos in her pool.

John Papalia, P.T., and Tom Lynn, P.T., helped with the medical aspects of the manuscript while coaches Bobby Kersee and Allan Hanckel shared their knowledge of training world-class athletes.

Maria Doest and Deborah McCormick applied their coaching eyes to the martial arts photos.

Speedo America supplied all the bathing suits.

Carolyn McDaniel, Susan Lawrence, and the rest of the staff of Huey's Athletic Network and the staff of Robert Forster Physical Therapy contributed in numerous ways during the many months it took to write this book.

Massage therapists Craig Benedict, Andrew Maksym, and Gary Ochman lowered Lynda Huey's stress levels.

Random House editor Olga Seham had a vision of the importance of this book and offered encouragement and editorial guidance.

Agent Jane Jordan Browne helped keep this book project moving at several critical junctures.

The models in the photos listed below graciously gave their time to this book and have used The Waterpower Workout and The Deep Waterpower Workout during their athletic or dance careers:

Rod Brower—Competed at 800 meters for the University of California at Irvine and now competes for Track West. A former model, Rod is now an information systems consultant.

LaReine Chabut—Actress/dancer LaReine is the lead instructor of Volume 5 for the award-winning "FIRM" exercise series available on video. A top athletic model, she is a spokeswoman for Nike shoes and cover model for *Shape* magazine.

Laurie Chapman—A UCLA distance runner, then UCLA assistant coach who also taught Waterpower Workout classes for Huey's Athletic Network. She now lives in San Diego and wins many road races for Santa Monica Track Club. Laurie helped create The Deep Waterpower Workout.

Gea Johnson—The 1990 NCAA champion in the heptathlon and a straight-A student at Arizona State University. Gea had the world-leading performance in her event in May 1992, but injury sidelined her during the Barcelona Olympics.

Jackie Joyner-Kersee—An NCAA All-American in track and basketball for UCLA, Jackie won a silver medal in the heptathlon in the 1984 Olympics, two gold medals (long jump and heptathlon) in the 1988 Olympics, and one gold (heptathlon) and one bronze (long jump) medal in the 1992 Olympics.

Jacqui and Bill Landrum—Dance teachers at the University of Southern California. Respected choreographers for both film and television. Their credits include *Great Balls of Fire, Basic Instinct, The Doors,* and *China Beach.* They choreographed an award-winning Jimi Hendrix music video of "Voodoo Child." The Landrums helped create the Dance-Specific Waterpower Workout, and gave generously of their time in editing that chapter.

Holly Reineman—A fitness buff who has not let nine knee surgeries compromise her fit body and bold enthusiasm.

Kate Schmidt—A three-time Olympian and former world record holder in the javelin. Kate has worked in water exercise and water therapy since 1985. Kate willingly shared her water training expertise. She further assisted as liaison with water equipment manufacturers.

Cybill Shepherd—At nineteen, Cybill began her film career with *The Last Picture Show.* She has appeared in numerous other feature films, starred in the TV series *Moonlighting,* and has recently written and produced the TV movie *Memphis,* and produced *Stormy Weathers.* Cybill graciously let us use her pool for a photo shoot.

Contents

The
Complete
Waterpower
Workout Book

Introduction
The Magic of Water

Water adds magic to any workout. The magic lies in water's **support** for the body (buoyancy), water's **resistance** to body movement, and water's wonderful **freshness**.

Buoyancy is the upward thrust exerted by water on a body that is totally or partially immersed in it. Water's buoyancy supports you as you move through it in a training program, letting you run, walk, leap, stretch, and pivot without the jolts that could cause injuries if these were done on land. Water acts as a cushion for your weight-bearing joints, preventing injury, strain, and reinjury common to other exercise programs.

At the same time that water supports the body, water resists movement through it. Any movement at any speed in any direction is slowed by water's resistance. Three-dimensional resistance is created as your body pushes the water out of its way. Because water is denser than air, your muscles work harder in water than if you were simply moving your arms and legs through air on land. Water is, in effect, a natural weight-training machine that is instantly adjustable: The harder you push and pull and kick in the water, the more resistance you meet from it.

On land, such resistance would raise your body's temperature. But water dissipates heat faster than air does, so water's freshness keeps your body cool and soothed as if by massage.

The Great Equalizer

One of the most magical features of water training is its versatility and universal applicability. Water is the great equalizer; everyone—from workout rookies to professional athletes, seniors to pregnant women—can use it and enjoy its benefits. You can enter a water-training program anywhere along the fitness continuum and train alongside people of all fitness levels. Doing the same exercises at the same time, you can each be challenged by working at your respective optimum speeds and depths of water. And more important for some, you don't even have to be able to swim.

You may not have exercised in months or even years, yet you can enter the water and begin immediately. (Check with your doctor before beginning any exercise program and follow the safety tips that appear on pages 31–32.) Even if you have injuries that disable you on land, you can move easily and with assurance in the water. You may be cross training for your sport; you may be losing excess weight for the first time in years. Whatever your level of interest and involvement, you will learn that water is a wonderful friend to have on your side. It can assist you all the way from rehabilitation to gold medals. Those who have injuries will want to read the entire book, then focus on the Water Healing chapters 7 through 12. Those who are without injuries can begin to improve their fitness immediately with The Waterpower Workout or The Deep Waterpower Workout. The chart on page 14 will help direct you to the appropriate starting point.

Water, Water Every Day

Overtraining has been cited as the number one problem faced by fitness enthusiasts today. Most people don't know how to recognize overtraining symptoms. They can include repetitive injuries, staleness in workouts, and failure to achieve realistic fitness goals. You can avoid the overtraining syndrome by using water wisely.

You can do a water workout every day without worrying about straining your muscles or joints. This makes water exercise a perfect activity for those who enjoy daily exercise but have experienced overtraining injuries in the past from daily workouts on land.

If you know you shouldn't run today because of a sore knee, train in the water instead. If your elbow hurts and you can't play racquetball, train in the water. You can even use water when you're feeling too weak or tired for your normal land-based activity. Begin slowly, and if your body genuinely needs rest, simply stretch, kick, and recover in the water. But because water soothes away pain and muscle soreness, don't be surprised if you start a gentle water recovery and find your energy so lifted that you can perform a full Waterpower Workout.

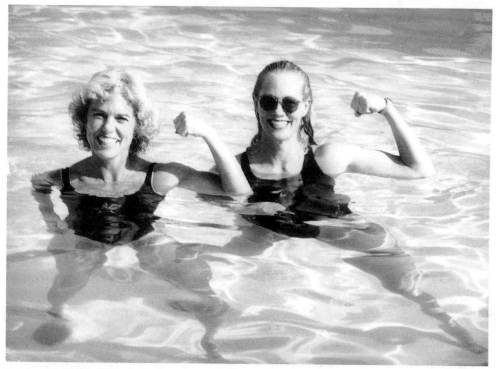

Lynda Huey and Cybill Shepherd have fun while they use Waterpower Workouts to stay in shape.

Where to Find Water

Some of you have pools in your backyards. Others have pools in their apartment building or condominium complex. But most of you have to go out and find a pool for your workout.

Nowadays nearly every community has a pool that can be used for a small fee. Your local college, YMCA, YWCA, YMHA, and recreation department are your best bets for finding inexpensive access to water. Health clubs charge more money but often have plusher facilities—sauna, steam room, Jacuzzi. Nearby hotels may offer swim memberships to the neighborhood.

Check your potential pool's schedule. Make sure there is a recreational swim time during which you can use the pool without interference from lap swimmers, children, or divers. Ideally, the pool you choose for your water training should be no more than ten to fifteen minutes from your home or from your workplace. The locker room should be clean, inviting, and comfortable. If your "home" pool is easily accessible, and if you are comfortable in its surroundings, you'll go more often than if it's unattractive or a long drive away. After you have found your home pool, don't stop looking for an extra water-training location, for your home pool may unexpectedly close for cleaning or the schedule may change, conflicting with your ideal training time. You should have op-

The Magic of
Water

5

tions, so locate at least one other possible site for water exercise. With approximately 6.5 million pools nationwide (6 million residential and a half million commercial) you should be able to find at least two to call your own.

When you travel, plan to stay at a hotel or motel that has a pool and use it. If a vacation takes you to a lake, calm river, or flat sea, do an open-water workout.

Private Tanks

With the recent explosion in water training and water rehabilitation, new options are being created for supplying the main ingredient: water. Single-person and small-group tanks are now available and being used in hospitals, therapy centers, and training rooms. Although originally designed for therapy, they provide anyone with the ideal small workout pool. Homes that housed private gyms are now housing private tanks for year-round water training. All have multiple-sectional design or are modular in construction, allowing them to go through most doorways for installation in preexisting rooms. Precautions should be taken to protect nonswimmers and children from drowning.

The **SwimEx** hydrotherapy system* is 17 feet, 6 inches long, 7 feet, 8 inches wide, and is available in models of three depths: 42 inches, 50 inches, and 60 inches. All are equipped with a paddlewheel propulsion system that creates a broad, controllable flow of water in over forty different speeds. (See Photo B.) Cross-training or injured athletes, fitness enthusiasts, and postsurgical patients can swim or run in place against this variable water resistance. Also, the angled surfaces around the bottom edge provide work stations for numerous total-body exercises. The 60-inch Multidepth model offers 10-inch and 15-inch floor inserts that change the water depth to 50 inches and 45 inches to accommodate people of all heights and abilities. Multiple depths provide options to train from total suspension through stages of increased weight bearing. The tank's installation requires less than 200 square feet.

The **Aquarius** rehabilitation tank's most popular size is 8 feet long, 8 feet wide, and 54 inches in depth, although other depths are also available. Made of stainless steel, it can be installed in a space 12 by 12 feet. An Aquarius water workout station (see page 100) is mounted on one wall of the pool. Handrails on the other walls allow for stretching, tethered running, and tethered swimming.

The **HydroWorx** standard model measures 10 feet long, 6 feet wide, and 8 feet deep. The movable floor can be lowered from the existing floor surface to as low as 10 feet depending on the HydroWorx model. Furthermore, the floor is actually a variable-speed, reversible treadmill with speeds ranging from a crawl to 10 mph. The floor is designed to provide the sensation of walking or running on moist sand. The HydroWorx is made of stainless steel and has adjustable handrails along the sides. There are three large jets on the front wall and sixty smaller jets on the side walls. (See Photo C.) The water temperature can be adjusted from 92 degrees to 76 degrees in eight hours.

*A list of all products and manufacturers appearing in the text can be found in the Appendix (page 359).

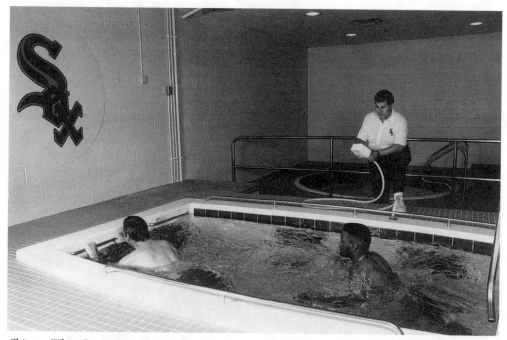

Chicago White Sox trainer Herm Schneider monitors water flow in Swimex for pitcher Charlie Hough and outfielder Tim Raines.

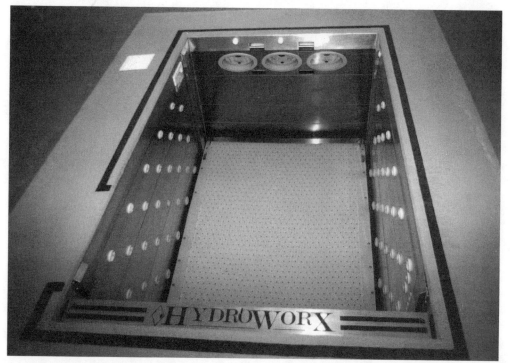

Small indoor pools like the HydroWorx are becoming increasingly popular in clinics and in people's homes.

The Magic of
Water

D

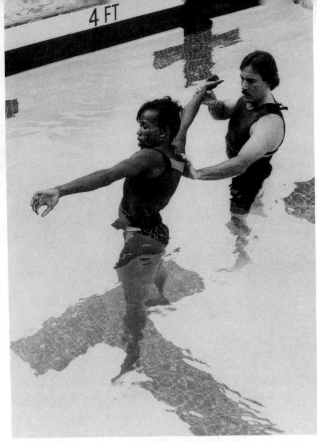

Robert Forster stretching Jackie Joyner-Kersee, who is wearing the Wet Wrap.

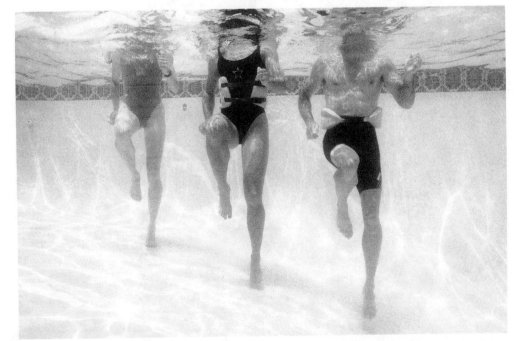

Low *impact shallow-water running (left),* **lower** *impact shallow-water running with Aqua Belt (middle), and* **no** *impact deep-water running with Wet Sweat Belt.*

Water Versatility

You can create a water workout in any size pool and within a wide range of temperatures. While tiny hotel and backyard pools are often too short for satisfying lap swimming, they are perfect for water training. As long as you can stretch out your arms and legs, the pool is big enough to serve as your water gym. If the water is warm (88 to 92 degrees), you can focus on improving your flexibility with water stretches or slowly begin the specific rehabilitation exercises of Water Healing. If the water temperature is moderate (82 to 87 degrees), you can comfortably perform all Waterpower and Deep Waterpower exercises either slowly or at high intensity depending upon your fitness level. If the water is cool (72 to 81 degrees), and you would become chilled if you didn't train hard and fast the entire water workout, wear **The Wet Wrap** for added warmth (see Photo D). This wet-suit vest is easier to use than traditional vests because it simply wraps around the body instead of being pulled over the head, and its adjustable strap lets you get a snug fit for the most warmth. The Wet Wrap comes in many colors and in all adult and children sizes.

Every pool has unique features, and if you familiarize yourself with steps, ladders, corners, and slants, you will soon learn to place each exercise in the exact location where it can best be performed. Kicking exercises work well with your back to a corner or when you sit on a step. Enhance stretches by grasping a ladder, gutter, or skimmer box with your hands. Running is best performed on either a flat surface or a downhill slant, while an uphill slant is fine for back kicks.

Most pools have both shallow and deep water. To add variety to your water training, learn exercise routines for both ends of the pool.

When you strap on a flotation device and begin deep-water exercise, you will find a challenging overall conditioning program with emphasis on the abdominal, back, shoulder, and upper thigh muscles. In deep water you experience a floating sensation and no impact to your weight-bearing joints, although you must expend more energy working on balance.

Standing in chest-deep water at the other end of the pool, you weigh only 10 percent of your normal body weight. So even the most powerful jumps conclude with a low-impact landing. Shallow-water training offers maximum muscular conditioning to the lower legs and provides precise simulation of dance and sports movement for cross-training purposes.

The Waterpower Workout appears in Chapter 2. The Deep Waterpower Workout follows in Chapter 3. If you have a lower-body injury or if you've been sedentary many years, start with The Deep Waterpower Workout for a month or two before moving to The Waterpower Workout. Or you may decide to stay in deep water simply because you enjoy it. Both deep and shallow workouts bring progress and fitness.

Athletes and dancers will want to bring specific skills into the pool for refinement. Chapters 4 and 5 illustrate how. Chapters 7 through 12 show those who are hurt how to protect their injury while following a progressive rehabilitation plan.

Whichever program you choose as your starting point, photocopy the photo summary at the end of that chapter. Laminate it or seal it in plastic and take it with you to the pool.

Comparison of Water and Land Training

Strong body alignment. Most people strengthen only the muscles at the front of the body, the ones they can see in the mirror: biceps, pectorals, quadriceps. Yet for daily life, it's even more important to strengthen the muscles at the back of the body, the ones that help fight gravity and ensure good postural alignment. In fact, most of the painful conditions that require therapeutic treatment are a result of stress placed on the body by poor posture. Therefore, you need to strengthen your "antigravity" muscles: trapezius, rhomboids, gluteals, hamstrings, and erector spinae. The Waterpower Workout is designed to strengthen these muscles, which hold you effortlessly in proper postural alignment.

Balanced strength in muscle pairs. Back-and-forth movements of the arms, legs, trunk, and even the eyes are possible only because muscles work in synchronized pairs—when one contracts, the opposing one relaxes. The muscles executing the actual movement are known as agonists. As the agonists contract, the opposing muscle group, the antagonists, must relax to allow movement to occur. Then in the returning movement the muscles reverse roles. This reciprocal contraction and relaxation continues, allowing for smooth, back-and-forth movement.

Muscle pairs maintain a specific ratio of strength to each other. If that ratio is thrown out of balance by training only one of the muscles in a pair, you produce inefficiency and the potential for injury. Therefore, it is extremely important to exercise both muscles of each antagonistic pair: quadriceps/hamstrings, biceps/triceps, abductors/adductors, and so forth.

Any exercise in water forces you to work both halves of each muscle pair. For every push forward against water's resistance, you must pull backward to the starting position. For every swing upward, you must swing downward. When you exercise in water, symmetry is built in. For instance, you work both the bicep and tricep with the same arm curl, because you meet resistance to your movement in both directions of the exercise. First the biceps contract to bend the elbow, then the triceps contract to extend the arm to a straight position. Just keep in mind that you must **work with equal force in both directions of movement** if you intend to keep balance in your muscle pairs.

Aerobic and anaerobic fitness. Aerobic fitness allows for moderate, continuous endurance exercise. Anaerobic fitness is necessary for strenuous bursts of speed and explosive power. Both aerobic and anaerobic fitness are vital to a well-conditioned person. A person who is aerobically fit has increased capacity to perform physical movements, has a more favorable ratio of good to bad cholesterol, has protection against many diseases, and has a stronger sense of well-being.

On land, continuous aerobic exercise can make your muscles feel heavy. An hour of running, aerobics, power walking, mountain biking, or rope jumping jolts the skeletal system. Land-based intensive interval training to build the body's anaerobic capacity is accompanied by extreme fatigue and impact to the muscles, connective tissues, and weight-bearing joints. In water, however, aerobic work is achieved effortlessly while anaerobic work sneaks in almost painlessly. Although you feel a sense of great strength against resistance, you finish the workout feeling fresh.

Increased flexibility. Although stretching is a peaceful and soothing activity for most people on land, for some it produces discomfort and strain. These people will benefit greatly from stretching in water, where comfort and relaxation are virtually built in. Nearly everyone will find stretching in water enjoyable, and enjoying stretching means you'll do it more often, for longer periods of time, and with more regularity. That adds up to faster progress.

Once you warm up and adapt to the initial chill of entering the water, your body begins to relax. In fact, it relaxes in water like nowhere else. When you're buoyed by water, the supportive role of your muscles is diminished and muscles can relax more easily. This relaxation promotes comfortable, rhythmic breathing, which aids your stretching. The calm sensation you work for while stretching on land comes almost automatically in the low-gravity environment of water.

Overall balance and coordination. In the Waterpower exercises, you will be forced to use your abdominal and back muscles as well as your arms and legs to maintain erect body alignment and balance. This improved balance will carry over into your sports and daily activities.

When you walk or run on land, your right arm and left leg move at the same time. This is called cross-crawl patterning. You learned it as a baby when you crawled on the ground. It takes no thought; it simply happens. In water, many people become disoriented to the opposition of their limbs, but water training increases coordination by virtue of its emphasis on cross-crawl patterning, which is the basis of all human coordination. By practicing moving your right arm at the same time as your left leg, and doing it against the resistance of water, you will improve your strength in these oppositional movements.

Once you've mastered moving in opposition, you'll find that all of your movements, in water and on land, are more coordinated. So **take time to develop smooth opposition movement patterns** on any exercise that causes problems.

The natural, rhythmic quality of water exercises plus the sensation of water's resistance will make you aware of any jerkiness or imbalance in your movements. As you work toward smoother movement and better balance in your water training, you will find yourself moving more gracefully with fewer extraneous movements on land.

A sense of well-being. What an amazing change in attitude we experience as soon as we enter the water! Stress washes away. Anger, disappointment, and aggravation go with it. The moment we become immersed in water, we have entered a new environment of sensation and perception. We can learn to use this quality of water to diffuse built-up negative emotions. No matter what seems to be going wrong, we can go to the water.

Rehabilitation

Most people turn to water for the first time during a crisis. Whatever the injury or disability that has led you to water, you will find that Water Healing Workouts soothe your body and mind. The moment you slide into the water for an emergency water workout, you feel significantly better. Pain is reduced; mobility is regained. Where you felt inability, now there is capability. Where you sensed helplessness, now there is hope. In water you can move, stretch, walk, and even run when all that seemed impossible on land. You can build a Water Healing Workout that protects the injured body part from further harm while the rest of the body continues to train. You will find that you regain, maintain, or actually improve strength and endurance.

Injury sites gradually heal and naturally begin reasserting themselves during Water Healing Workouts. As though they had a mind of their own, the formerly injured areas begin handling more weight, more impact, more speed. Water Healing becomes more strenuous, crossing over into Waterpower, preparing for the return to land. Water can be our most helpful companion and healing partner for life.

To Gold Medals

An athlete's worst nightmare comes true when fitness is at its peak and injury strikes. The frustration of unfulfilled promise is heartbreaking and the agony of inactivity is often worse than the pain of the injury itself. So when injured athletes find an environment in which to continue their high-pitched training and not lose that sharply honed edge, they feel great relief. They use The Deep Waterpower Workout, The Waterpower Workout, and Sport-Specific Waterpower Workouts to hasten their return to land without losing fitness.

Although most world-class athletes, like their nonathletic peers, usually turn to water the first time during a crisis, the wise ones learn to use this valuable training tool as a preventative measure as well. No longer will they "force" a workout when joint or muscle pain says to take a day off. Now they immediately turn to water and take a day off without taking a day off. Instead of pounding the pavement twice a day, seven days a week, distance runners often do several of their long runs in deep water. Instead of sprinting on the synthetic track five days in a row, Olympic speedsters often substitute one of their weekly workouts with sprints in water. Professional football, soccer, tennis, and basketball players have recently begun taking the plunge too. Like professional and Olympic athletes, you can avoid strain and injury while moving closer to your fitness goals by letting water work its magic for you.

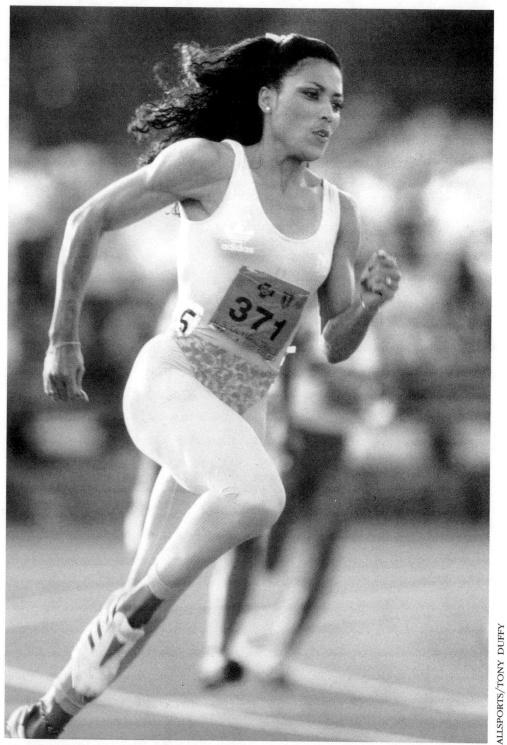

*Florence Griffith Joyner used The Waterpower Workout to retain her form and speed during a
hamstring injury.*

Where to Begin

Fitness Level	Goals	Start With
Beginner		
Inactive for years	Increased strength	DW
Overweight	Weight loss	DW
Afraid of water	Increased balance	WP
Elderly	Increased flexibility	WD/DW/WP
Pregnant	Improved aerobic capacity	WD/DW/WP
Fitness Enthusiast		
Conditioning program in progress	Improved aerobic/anaerobic capacity	WP/DW
	Increased muscular strength	WP/DW
	Weight control	WP/DW
Training Athlete or Dancer		
All sports or ballet	Superior aerobic/anaerobic capacity	PH/WP/DW
	Superior muscular strength	WP
	Increase in speed and power	PH/WP
	Prevention of injuries	WD/DW/WP
	Increased flexibility	WD/DW/WP
	Improvement in skill	SS or DS
Injured Athlete or Dancer	Acceleration of healing time	WH/DW
	Retention of top fitness	DW/WP
	Little loss of skill	SS/DS/WP
	Quick return to sport or dance	SS/DS/WP
Presurgical Patient		
Training prior to surgery	Gain top possible fitness, decrease postsurgical loss of fitness	WH/DW/WP
Postsurgical Patient		
Recovering from surgery, accident, or illness	Regain strength, balance	WH/DW
	Regain mobility, coordination	WH/DW
	Increased flexibility	WH/DW/WP

WP = The Waterpower Workout
DW = The Deep Waterpower Workout
WH = Water Healing Workout
SS = Sport-Specific Waterpower Workout

DS = Dance-Specific Waterpower Workout
WD = The Waterpower Warm-Down
PH = The Twenty-five-Minute Powerhouse Workout

I

Waterpower

Designing Your Water Fitness Program

Although it is generally understood that a high level of fitness is necessary to participate in athletics, most people don't realize that a certain level of fitness is required just to perform daily tasks. Greater fitness levels translate into improved performance for the marathon, the weekend softball game, or unloading the groceries from the car.

What is fitness and how do you attain it?

The Nine Aspects of Fitness

The word *fitness* itself is difficult to define in a single synonym or even a long-winded paragraph. But there are nine key aspects of fitness: flexibility, aerobic and anaerobic capacity, musculoskeletal resiliency, strength, power, speed, skills, and rest. With a greater understanding of these fitness components you will be able to construct a personal program that helps you overcome your physical shortcomings and improves upon your strengths.

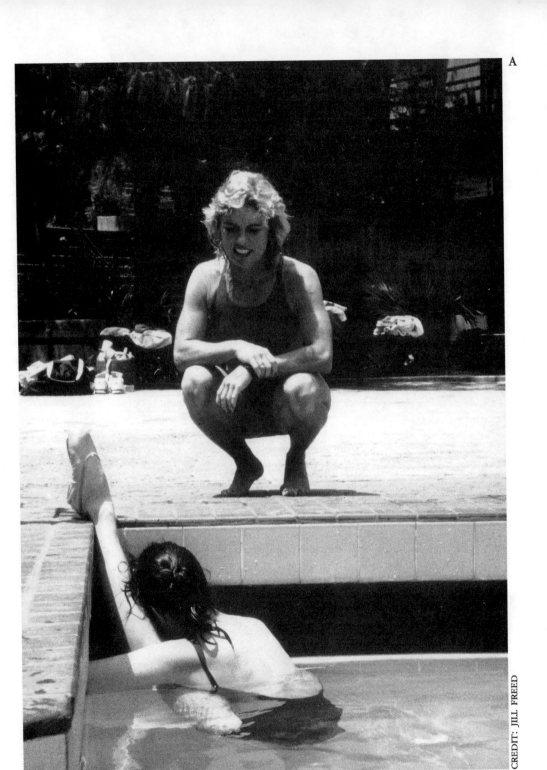

Dancers and athletes use Waterpower for cross training. Here, Lynda Huey helps dancer Melissa Lesly work on flexibility.

Flexibility is the range of motion of a body part as it moves around a joint. Increased range of motion allows for more efficient movement and fewer injuries. Although it is commonly thought that muscles are the limiting factor in flexibility, it is, in fact, the connective tissue surrounding muscle fibers and making up tendons (which attach muscles to bone), ligaments (which connect bones at a joint), and fasciae (which provide support to muscles) that limit movement. Muscles are inherently elastic. They relax as you stretch. The stretch is then passed along to the real target of your flexibility work: the connective tissue. **Take advantage of water's soothing qualities to work with determination on your flexibility.**

Aerobic capacity is the body's ability to perform activity for extended periods of time. Aerobic fitness improves the body's ability to deliver oxygen to the working muscles. On one end of this system the heart becomes stronger and on the other a better network of capillaries (the smallest blood vessels) infiltrates muscles, bringing oxygen and nutrients closer to the actual working muscle cell. But the greatest (and widely unrecognized) improvement in fitness occurs within the muscle cells themselves. The aerobic enzyme systems are housed there; they are responsible for combining oxygen with nutrients to make energy for muscle contraction. These aerobic enzyme systems, made more efficient through physical training, provide continuous fuel for continuous work periods. Because these enzyme systems use fat as their fuel, aerobically fit people have higher fat-burning capability. In effect, their muscles have become more efficient "fat-burning factories." With proper diet, this leads to leaner, healthier bodies.

Improvements in heart efficiency come with exercise. The heart, answering the demands of the working muscles, becomes a stronger and more efficient pump. The American College of Sports Medicine states that in order to experience an aerobic training effect, you must achieve a working heart rate that is continuously elevated to your "target heart rate zone," twenty to sixty minutes each workout, three to five times a week. Your target heart rate for aerobic benefit is 65 to 85 percent of your maximum heart rate. Maximum heart rates can be exactly determined with treadmill stress tests or you can use the predicted rates in the chart on page 51 based on national norms for your age and sex. Moderate, continuous training such as this takes the body to a "steady state" of aerobic exercise that requires an elevated but comfortable breathing pattern. **Aerobic exercise is most easily accomplished in water where you are cooled and hardly feel a change in your breathing rate.**

Anaerobic capacity is the body's ability to perform work without oxygen. When exercise becomes severe, the body's aerobic systems can no longer provide enough oxygen to meet the demands of the muscles. The point where the body switches to its anaerobic (without oxygen) systems is called the anaerobic threshold. When exercise is performed in the anaerobic state, complicated chemical processes take place in muscle tissue, allowing muscle contraction to continue in spite of the absence of oxygen. Anaerobic work creates an "oxygen debt"—the amount of oxygen needed to process the waste products produced during anaerobic muscle contraction. This oxygen debt must be paid back at the completion of exercise, which explains why the heart rate and breathing remain elevated following an intense workout. Interval training that primarily calls for anaerobic work with recovery intervals allows you to push back your anaerobic threshold so that more can be accomplished in the aerobic state and you can "pay as you go," avoiding oxygen debt. **Anaerobic work can be performed in the water without the muscle and joint strain that occurs on land.**

Musculoskeletal resiliency (MSR) is the strength of the bones and the connective tissue that makes up tendons, ligaments, and surrounds muscles. When a muscle contracts, force is transmitted through the tendon, which pulls on the bone, causing movement. These tendon-bone junctures are subject to stress and are often the site of strain and injury. Conversely, the same sites become stronger with appropriate stimulus—force that is not great enough to strain the connective tissue or injure the bone. Additional connective tissue is deposited in areas of stress, and even bones become stronger as greater calcium is deposited within the bone cells due to training stimulus. These adaptive processes can become overburdened, however, if work load is inappropriately difficult for an athlete's present condition. The result is injury. Be aware, however, that MSR is sport specific. Just because your knees have been made resilient to the demands of running doesn't necessarily mean they have been adequately toughened for the specific demands of mountain biking. Thus you must plan to build your MSR for each activity you undertake. **Maintain musculoskeletal resilience with continuous water training; never take more than ten consecutive days of complete rest.**

Strength is a muscle's ability to exert force. Adequate strength allows for proper body mechanics in everyday living and for improved athletic performance. Increased muscular strength allows athletes to kick and hit harder and throw farther while it permits endurance athletes to use a smaller percentage of available muscle fibers to complete each running step, each swimming stroke, or each cycling revolution, thereby leaving more rested muscle fibers for recruitment later in the competition. The result is greater efficiency. Stronger muscles are less likely to be strained. Further, they provide good protection against joint injury. **Use some of the resistance equipment demonstrated throughout the book to quickly gain strength.**

Power is force times velocity (speed). How fast a muscle exerts force against any object or against the ground translates into power. In sport, power is probably more important than absolute strength. Power is developed by resistive exercise at a high speed, or with jumping or bounding drills (plyometrics). **Performing drills in water rather than on land makes this elusive component of fitness more easily attainable and less likely to cause injury.**

Speed is the rate of a limb's movement around a joint. The coordination of movements occurring at several joints translates into higher speed (velocity of movement). Today's advanced coaching methods develop speed by breaking down a given sport skill into its component movements and strengthening the primary muscles involved in performing each of them. Then, the strengthened movements are reassembled into a faster execution of the whole skill. **Training for speed is done equally well on land and in water, but has proven less injurious in water.**

Skills are neuromuscular habit patterns that allow athletes to perform their activities with efficiency. Some sports demand many high-level skills—for example, baseball, tennis, ice skating, and gymnastics. Athletes in these sports must learn, then master and be able to duplicate on demand, precise throws, swings, hits, jumps, spins, slides, and flips.

Establishing habit patterns of such skills takes hundreds and hundreds of repetitions and long hours of practice. Runners, cyclists, and swimmers, who do virtually the same single movement again and again, also need to devote time to establish their best possible form and efficiency, then to keep it sharp throughout the year. **Water's density requires more deliberate performance of sports movements, giving athletes and coaches the perfect opportunity to correct or improve skills.**

Rest is an integral part of every training program, for Olympians and recreational athletes alike. The body adapts to work stimulus only if a rest period follows.
Remember:

$$\text{STRESS} \quad + \quad \text{RECOVERY TIME} \quad = \quad \text{ADAPTATION}$$
$$\text{(Exercise)} \qquad\qquad \text{(Rest)} \qquad\qquad \text{(Fitness Gains)}$$

The above equation dictates that athletes follow the **Hard/Easy Principle** of training. Each hard workout should be followed by an easy workout to allow for adaptation to take place. One hard workout followed by another (stress plus more stress) often equals breakdown, staleness, or poor performance. Within each month's plan, there should be one easier work week as well. **By moving a low-intensity version of your sport into the water, you can create an active-rest water workout.**

Fitness Training Variables

Always keep in mind the nine aspects of fitness above as you build your water-training program. Keep in mind also these three important training variables:

Frequency. To achieve systematic progress in your training program you must complete a minimum of three workouts a week. **Those who train *only* in water can work out up to six days per week as long as they program at least two *easier* Waterpower Workouts each week.** For those two workouts, do fewer repetitions and take longer rests between water exercises.

Intensity. Your working heart rate (see page 51) is the primary means of measuring how hard you are exercising—the intensity of your workout. Heart rate is an objective measure of intensity, but there is also a subjective one called perceived rate of exertion. As they train, participants ask themselves, "Are my lungs and muscles burning as I water walk a fast one-minute interval? Are my arms and legs pushing through the water at 50, 75, or 90 percent of max?" However, this measure of perceived exertion is not as precise as measuring heart rate, because the average person doesn't know how a 100 percent effort feels in order to estimate a lower percentage rate of exertion. But as you work at higher levels and become more experienced in training, you will become better able to gauge the intensity of your workout.

Volume. The number of sets and repetitions you do during a weight-training session, the number of miles you swim or run, the number of swings you take at a baseball or kicks at a football—this is volume, a training variable. Reps refers to the number of times in a row you repeat a given exercise. When you complete a series of reps, you have finished your first set. If you were to do a second set, you would begin after a specified rest period.

Intensity and volume are inversely related: To complete high-intensity workouts, the volume must be low; to do a greater volume of work, the intensity must be low. Volume lays the foundation of performance while intensity brings about the athlete's top performance level.

In building your water-training program, you must consider all three of these variables, trying to achieve a balance among them that will progress your fitness improvements while avoiding injury and overtraining. By using the concept of periodization in your training, which dictates how to manipulate these variables, you will scientifically build your fitness in preparation for maximum performance.

Periodization of Training

Whether you are a professional athlete, a fitness enthusiast, or a sports rookie, planning your **yearly training program** will assure you of rapid and consistent progress. **Each season will have specific goals,** and thus wherever you are in your yearly training cycle, **each workout you do will have a purpose**.

Elite athletes have taught us the principles of periodization in training programs. **Periodization is the rational organization of the training cycle to achieve opti-**

B

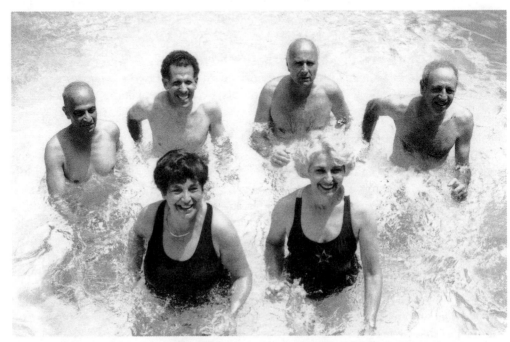

Waterpower helps people of all ages look better and feel better. This group water-trains only.

mal development of all aspects of fitness. Periodization dictates that the year be broken into an early season, a transition season, a peak performance (competition) season, then an active rest season. Within each season the training variables—frequency of exercise, intensity of exercise, and volume of exercise—are manipulated in specific workouts for desired results. Each yearly schedule ends with an active rest that allows the body to recover in preparation for the next year's cycle.

You may decide to make Waterpower and Deep Waterpower your primary exercise for fitness. In this case, fitness gains are best achieved by varying the interval training segments of your water workouts. Interval training, performed in both deep and shallow water, is intermittent exercise that consists of high-intensity work periods broken up with specified rest periods. As you move through the seasons of your yearly plan, the length and intensity of your intervals will change. Chapters 2 and 3 explain how to progress from Level 1 to Level 2 of Waterpower and Deep Waterpower workouts, which you will do as you move from early season to the transition season. As the year passes, you will work your way to Level 3 and achieve your peak fitness level for the year.

You may decide to fit Waterpower into your existing cross-training program that now includes running and weight training, or cycling and basketball, or racquetball, yoga, and rock climbing, or another combination of workouts. If you do, the easiest and safest way to proceed is to replace one or two of your land workouts each week with Waterpower. As you do so, consider the training variables and periodization of training principles set forth in this chapter.

Your Yearly Plan

Each of the four seasons of the yearly training cycle has a specific role in developing the nine aspects of fitness (see page 17).

Early season. This season lasts eight to fourteen weeks, during which a fitness base must be established. With the use of low-intensity exercises, the body is stressed to a degree that stimulates an increase of **aerobic capacity** and **musculoskeletal resiliency**. The theme during this season is to start slowly with low volume, low intensity and build higher volume and only moderate intensity. **Flexibility** exercises are also emphasized at this time because they assist in developing musculoskeletal resiliency while they also help create the range of motion needed for proper biomechanics, or form. **Skill** development begins here with slow drills designed to lay a framework of coordination.

If you are water training only, build your base during this season by doing two Waterpower Workouts and two Deep Waterpower Workouts at Level 1 each week. During the early season, consider The Waterpower Workout as a hard workout in the hard/easy scheme of training. Consider The Deep Waterpower Workout easy in your plan, because it is less stressful on your joints and allows for maximum recovery even while it continues to challenge your fitness level. Continue with this plan a total of two to three months. Emphasize water stretching.

Cross-training athletes must carefully and slowly build an early-season base on land, but they can work in water at a slightly higher intensity. Do one Waterpower Workout

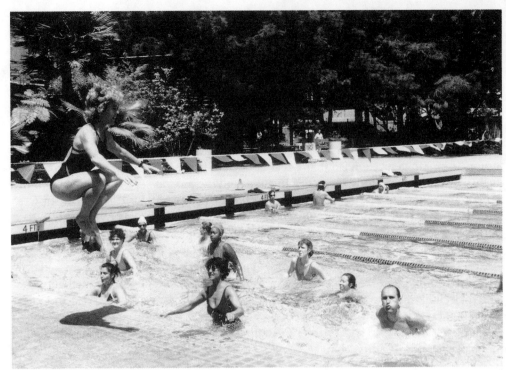

Plyometrics such as explosive jumps and leaps can be done by virtually everyone in water, when most people couldn't do them on land.

and one Deep Waterpower Workout at Level 2 each week through the entire early season, adding your sport-specific exercises (Chapter 5). Practice the hard/easy principle of training by breaking up back-to-back land workouts with Waterpower (Day 1 = land; Day 2 = water; Day 3 = land) or use Waterpower as your second workout of the day following your easiest land days. Intervals should include two to three 3-minute runs and one to two 5-minute runs. Begin skill drills in water. Perform progressively larger volumes of low-intensity skill drills for eight to fourteen weeks.

Transition season. After building a base of aerobic fitness, musculoskeletal resiliency, and flexibility in the early season, but before full-blown competition begins, athletes must pass through a transition season. This eight- to fourteen week season prepares athletes for the specific rigors of their event while further improving their **aerobic and anaerobic capacity**. The major new emphasis of this season is a gradual increase in the intensity of workouts to develop first **strength**, then **power**. The volume of work plateaus through this season as the intensity builds. Within a workout you can perform greater intensities of exercise by breaking down the total work into short sprints interspersed with rest periods.

   The Waterpower workouts of the first three to four weeks in this season include strength work. During the final three to four weeks of transition, you must develop power by emphasizing high-intensity, explosive exercises. By nature these exercises are stressful to the body, which makes this critical transitional season the most difficult to achieve on land without suffering injury. Many athletes simply do too much too soon and their bodies break down. Avoid this by maintaining your hard/easy scheme and by integrating more Waterpower Workouts into your program. For in water you are cushioned in your explosive jumps, bounds, and hops; therefore, you can develop power more effectively and safely than on land. The body's musculoskeletal resiliency must be increased gradually to tolerate these higher loads of impact; the connective tissues and bone must be strengthened to accept greater stresses as muscles and joints move with more speed and power. By performing many repetitions of your plyometric power moves in water, you can later move to land with the confidence that you are prepared to handle the jolts of impact. Thus Waterpower plays an increasingly vital role in the transitional season of all land-based athletes.

If you are water training only, start your transition season by moving to the Level 2 program and performing two to three Waterpower Workouts and two to three Deep Waterpower Workouts each week. Your intervals should consist of fast runs from thirty seconds to two minutes. This program will further tax your aerobic and anaerobic capacities. To increase strength, add resistance equipment—Speedo SwimMitt XTs, Wave Webs, SpaBells, the Aquatoner, or Hydro-Tone bells—when you perform arm exercises 25 through 29 (pages 61 through 65). Use the Aquatoner or Hydro-Tone boots for leg exercises 31, 32, 34, and 35 (pages 67 through 69, 71 and 72). The equipment dramatically increases the force you must exert to move through the water, so move slowly at first to avoid muscle or tendon strain. (Descriptions of equipment appear in Chapters 3 (pages 85 and 86) and 8 (pages 230, 231, and 234), and in the Appendix (page 359).

Three to four weeks into the season, increase your number of repetitions of power exercises—the jumps, bounds, and kicks—and focus on the height of each jump and the speed of each leg and arm.

Cross-training athletes can begin performing *all* exercises against added resistance. Wear Speedo SwimMitts throughout the entire program, significantly increasing the work load of the arms, shoulders, back, and chest.

When you move to the power segment of this transitional season, focus on height of all jumping exercises and speed of all leg- and arm-swinging movements. Before you try any of your power (plyometric) drills on land, perform many repetitions in the water. Duplicate the technique and posture as accurately in water as you can.

Spend at least eight to fourteen weeks moving cautiously through this transition season before attempting any serious performance in your event. If you wish to begin distance racing, for example, remember that the emphasis is on building, not peaking, so don't set unrealistic goals too early. Simply use your twice-monthly 10-kilometer road race or 30-kilometer bike race as motivation. Intervals during this season should include four to six 30-second water sprints or three to four 2-minute sprints.

Skill development continues, adding speed to these drills, focusing on accuracy and precision.

Peak season. The first two seasons in your annual training program developed your base for physiological performance. Your goal during the next season—**peak fitness** or **competition**—is to sharpen your **skills** and improve your **speed** while maintaining

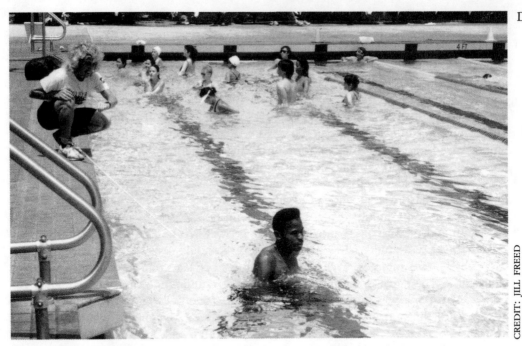

Olympic gold medalist Danny Everett runs in water whenever sore after competition.

the work you have already accomplished. It takes four weeks to reach your peak and this can only be maintained for approximately eight to twelve weeks.

Desire and motivation are key components in moving up from the base you've built to the peak. Sustain that motivation by appreciating the hard work you've already accomplished. Notice how your body has changed and how much easier the exercises seem even though you are pushing harder against the water and performing more repetitions. Feel how your clothes fit you differently, how the curves of newly developed muscles have brought sleeker lines to your body. Observe your new eating habits: Because you are always preparing for a workout, you make better food choices. Your body begins to dictate healthier foods at mealtime. You not only look good but you feel terrific.

Water trainers will move to Level 3 in your program and work hard with concentration on each exercise four to six times per week. Alternate between The Waterpower and Deep Waterpower workouts as you choose. Use short sprint intervals of forty-five seconds or less. Run them as fast as you can. Count how many arm strokes you can perform in ten seconds. Each right-left cycle equals one stroke: A twenty-stroke count is good; twenty-five is superior; thirty is excellent.

Try running intervals up to two minutes in length only if you can sustain at least 90 percent of your top speed.

During this competition season, cross-training athletes perform less endurance and strength work and focus instead on maintaining power and honing skills. Workouts that contain such power training and high-level skill work are high intensity. Therefore, frequency of workouts must be diminished. Use The Waterpower Warm-Down immediately after hard land workouts or the day between hard workouts to promote recovery and to allow your body to adapt to the increased intensity of peak-season training. Athletes who have difficulty maintaining high-intensity land workouts without injury can replace some of their land workouts with the high-intensity, low-stress Level 3 Deep Waterpower Workout, Level 3 of the Waterpower Workout, or the Twenty-five-Minute Powerhouse Workout. Insert short, fast intervals: six to eight 10-second sprints, four to six 20-second sprints, or three maximum-effort 45-second sprints.

The result is that with proper rest just prior to the event, an athlete is fully prepared for maximum performance on schedule. Enjoy these months of peak performance, but remember that you can't sustain this peak for long. Soon you will move past this cycle into the active rest season of the off season.

Rest season. The active rest season lasts four to six weeks. Whether you are a competitor or a fitness enthusiast, a cross trainer or a water athlete only, whether you have met your goals for the year or not—it is now time to **rest**. Your body requires rest to replenish energy stores and to rebuild areas suffering from the microtrauma caused by continuous training, that is, repetitive stress that can lead to a cumulative injury. This is the time you have programmed into your yearly training cycle for emotional and mental recovery as well. Give yourself a break, look back over the year, and rejoice in your successes while taking note of your mistakes and weaknesses. Think about changes for the coming year.

But don't stop training altogether. There's a vast difference between reduced training and no training. Fitness continues as long as some training continues, but it vanishes quickly when training ceases; hence the term *active rest*. Stay active in low-intensity sports you enjoy and emphasize stretching, both in and out of the water.

Cross-training athletes should continue with these reduced workouts for four to six weeks, water trainers for four weeks. Don't feel guilty. Recent research concludes that aerobic fitness and improved heart function can be maintained during brief periods of up to a two-thirds reduction in training. Relax and have faith in your fitness.

Water trainers should mix up levels 1, 2, and 3, doing at least two workouts a week. Or take a month away from the pool so your return to Waterpower will be refreshing. Try yoga, tennis, mountain biking, kayaking, roller-skating, or backpacking.

Cross-training athletes should do one Level 1 Waterpower, one Level 1 Deep Water-power, and one Waterpower Warm-Down each week in addition to doing low-key, enjoyable activities. Go hiking, biking, walking, bowling, or relax more deeply than before in yoga classes. This sounds like a lot on paper, but will indeed be a rest compared to the rigors of competition.

If you are a landlocked athlete during most of the year, the rest season is a perfect time to introduce this valuable training medium to your yearly training cycle.

During your active rest season, you can begin thinking about your new yearly plan. You will start once again at the early season, building a base for more difficult work to follow. Master athletes (over forty) will try to continue matching performances of previous years, but some decline is natural due to the aging process. Younger athletes and fitness enthusiasts will usually start each year's early-season work at a higher level than last year's. In this way progression is made over the years.

You have now completed your yearly training cycle from start to end. You are at the forefront of scientific fitness training.

Water Training Only

Season	Training Variables	Fitness Goals Emphasized	Programs	Level
Early Season (8 to 14 weeks)	Frequency: 4/week Volume: Steadily increases Intensity: Low	Aerobic capacity Musculoskeletal resiliency Flexibility Learn proper form for all exercises (skill)	2 WP/week 2 DW/week Intervals: 1 to 3 minutes	1 1
Transition (8 to 14 weeks)	Frequency: 4 to 6/week Volume: Increases Intensity: Steadily builds	Aerobic capacity Anaerobic capacity Strength Power (add resistance equipment) Continued skill development	2 to 3 WP/week 2 to 3 DW/week Intervals: 30 seconds to 2 minutes	2 2
Peak Fitness (12 to 16 weeks)	Frequency: 4 to 6/week Volume: Increases Intensity: High	Anaerobic capacity Musculoskeletal resiliency Strength Power (use resistance equipment) Speed	2 to 3 WP/week 1 PH/week 2 to 3 DW/week Intervals: 10 seconds to 2 minutes (counting arm strokes)*	3 3
Active Rest (4 to 6 weeks)	Frequency: 2/week Volume: Reduced Intensity: Lower	Rest and recovery Healing Flexibility No equipment	1 WP/week 1 DW/week 1 WD after biking or hiking No intervals	1,2, or 3 1,2, or 3

*Explained in text

WP = The Waterpower Workoutt
DW = The Deep Waterpower Workout

WD = The Waterpower Warm-Down
PH = The Twenty-five-Minute Powerhouse Workout

Cross-Training Athletes

Season	Training Variables	Fitness Goals Emphasized	Programs	Level
Early Season (8 to 14 weeks)	Frequency: 2/week Volume: Gradually increasing Intensity: Low	Aerobic capacity Musculoskeletal resiliency Flexibility	1 WP + SS/week 1 DW/week Intervals: 3 to 5 minutes	2 2
Begin skill development				
Transition (8 to 14 weeks)	Frequency: 3/week Volume: Increasing Intensity: Increasing	Aerobic capacity Anaerobic capacity Strength Power (do water plyometrics; add resistance equipment) Continued skill development	1 WP + SS/week 1 DW + SS/week 1 WD/week Intervals: 30 seconds to 2 minutes	3 3
Competition (8 to 16 weeks)	Frequency: 2 to 3/week Volume: Plateau Intensity: High	Speed Fine-tuned skills Power Strength	2 WD/week after workouts 1 WP or DW/week, midweek 1 PH/week including water plyometrics WP replaces any workout where injury suspected Intervals: 10 to 45 seconds (counting arm strokes)*	 3
Active Rest (4 to 6 weeks)	Frequency: 3/week Volume: Reduced Intensity: Low	Rest and Recovery Healing of injuries Flexibility	1 WP/week 1 DW/week 1 WD after biking or hiking No intervals	1 or 2 1 or 2

*Explained in text

WP = The Waterpower Workout
DW = The Deep Waterpower Workout
SS = Sport-Specific Waterpower Workout

WD = The Waterpower Warm-Down
PH = The Twenty-five-Minute Powerhouse Workout

T w o

The Waterpower Workout ®

Y ou are ready to enter the water to achieve fitness, high-level training, healing, or other goals you have for yourself.

If you are not injured, begin either The Waterpower Workout in this chapter or The Deep Waterpower Workout in Chapter 3. It's your choice.

If you are injured, read chapters 2 and 3, then chapters 7 through 11, which present all exercises as well as a formula for designing your own personal Water Healing Workout. Consult the chart on page 14 to determine exactly where to begin.

Whether injured or not, always check with your doctor before beginning an exercise program.

The Waterpower Workout program has been taught with only a few variations since 1984 and has continuously provided a satisfying and effective workout for all ages, sizes, and fitness levels. In it, you will discover exercises that provide you with a solid aerobic and anaerobic workout, rounded out with exercises specifically for your abdominals, arms, shoulders, chest, back, and legs. These thirty-eight exercises take about forty-five minutes to complete. If time is short, and you are already fairly fit, perform the Twenty-five-Minute Powerhouse Workout, which begins on page 78.

On land you would need a lengthy warm-up stretch before attempting the jumps and sprints to follow. But because the water's resistance doesn't allow the body to work as fast as on land, and because the water provides a cushion for the explosive moves to come, there's much less risk of injury and thus less need for a lengthy warm-up before beginning The Waterpower Workout.

Adapt The Waterpower Workout to your fitness level by changing the speed of your movements or by moving into slightly deeper or slightly shallower water. If you're just getting started or aren't in very good shape, do Level 1 in shoulder-deep water and move slowly. If you're in reasonable shape, do Level 2 at a comfortable pace while applying a moderate amount of resistance against chest-deep water. Those in top shape can jump high and move fast through Level 3 in chest-deep water for a high-octane workout.

Tips for Safe and Enjoyable Waterpower Workouts

- If you are alone in a pool, make sure someone is nearby in case of emergency. Always use the "buddy system" whenever you exercise in open water—river, bay, ocean, or lake. If you can't find a friend to join you, have someone watch from shore. If you aren't familiar with the water's currents, surface, texture of the bottom, or possible underwater obstacles, ask a local resident or lifeguard about possible dangers *before* you enter the water. If you wish, you can modify some of the exercises, working against currents or waves to make them more difficult. In rocky areas, wear a pair of water-training shoes.

- Don't drink alcohol before a water workout. Alcohol impairs your balance, coordination, and judgment, and it alters your body's physiological response to exercise.

- Wait at least two to three hours after a big meal before starting a hard workout. If your workout is gentle (Level 1 or The Waterpower Warm-Down), you can decrease the waiting time to one hour.

- Most pools are cool, so as soon as you slide into the water, begin jogging or bouncing for a warm-up. Bouncing is a rhythmic up-and-down movement in which your knees bend, then straighten, then bend again.

- When you bounce or jump, inhale at the height of the jump and exhale at the lowest point near the water. This prevents you from accidentally swallowing water.

- Move to a spot in the pool where you can stand in chest-deep water and can extend your arms fully without hitting any obstacle, a swimmer, or another water exerciser.

- To avoid blisters on your toes or on the balls of your feet, find a pool with a friendly bottom surface or buy some water-training shoes.

- Begin the exercises slowly. If your body feels strong and energetic, increase the pace of the movements as well as the height of the jumps. If you feel tired, move more slowly and sit lower in the water. Don't be surprised if your body changes the way it feels midway through the workout: Obey it.

- If you are a nonswimmer, consider joining a class to learn to swim. You will feel safer each time you enter the water.

LEVEL 1

Follow the Level 1 program if you are pregnant, have not exercised for six months or longer if you are beginning the early season in your training program, or if you're recovering from surgery, an injury, or childbirth.

Sets and repetitions: Do one set of fourteen reps of each exercise.

Frequency: Two to three days a week.

To progress: Add reps up to twenty. Progress to Level 2.

LEVEL 2

Follow the Level 2 program if you have been participating in aerobic exercise regularly two to three days a week for four months or longer.

Sets and repetitions: Do one set of twenty reps of each exercise.

Frequency: Three to four days a week.

To progress: Add reps up to thirty. Progress to Level 3.

LEVEL 3

Follow the Level 3 program if you have been participating regularly in aerobic and anaerobic activity three to four days a week for six months or longer.

Sets and repetitions: Do one set of thirty reps of each exercise. Finish with an extra set of thirty reps of back kicks, leg swings, and bicycling.

Frequency: Four to six days a week.

To progress: When this level becomes comfortable, increase power: Jump higher and move faster.

Begin with a five-minute warm-up of running and bouncing across the shallow end of the pool. If you have a sore ankle, foot, shin, knee, hip, or back, put on a flotation belt. Wearing it throughout The Waterpower Workout reduces impact on your weight-bearing joints.

The primary muscle movers are listed for each exercise. The first muscle group listed is called upon most; the muscle groups that follow are listed in descending order of importance. Refer to the muscle chart on pages 34 and 35 for a better understanding of which muscles you'll be working. Since the gastrocnemius and the muscles of the feet are prime movers in exercises 1 through 17, they are not mentioned to avoid repetition. The abdominal and erector spinae muscles act as stabilizing muscles for the body in nearly all exercises, but are listed only in the exercises where they are prime movers.

BASIC MUSCLE GROUPS (front)

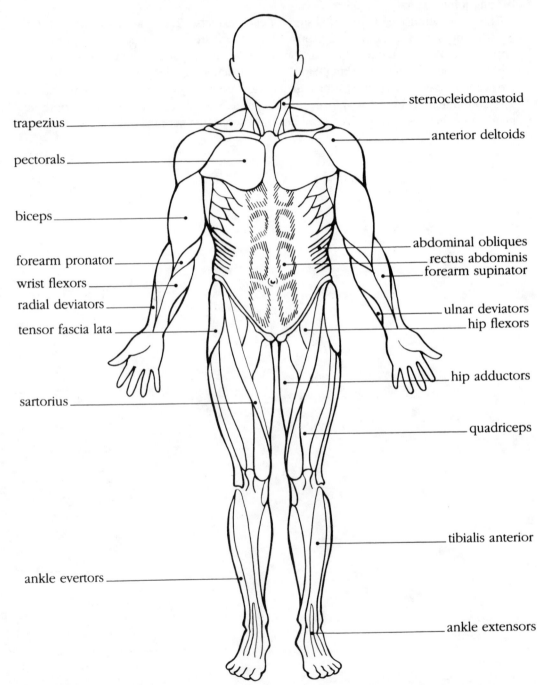

sternocleidomastoid

trapezius

anterior deltoids

pectorals

biceps

abdominal obliques
rectus abdominis
forearm supinator

forearm pronator

wrist flexors

radial deviators

ulnar deviators
hip flexors

tensor fascia lata

hip adductors

sartorius

quadriceps

tibialis anterior

The
Complete
Waterpower
Workout
Book

ankle evertors

ankle extensors

BASIC MUSCLE GROUPS (back)

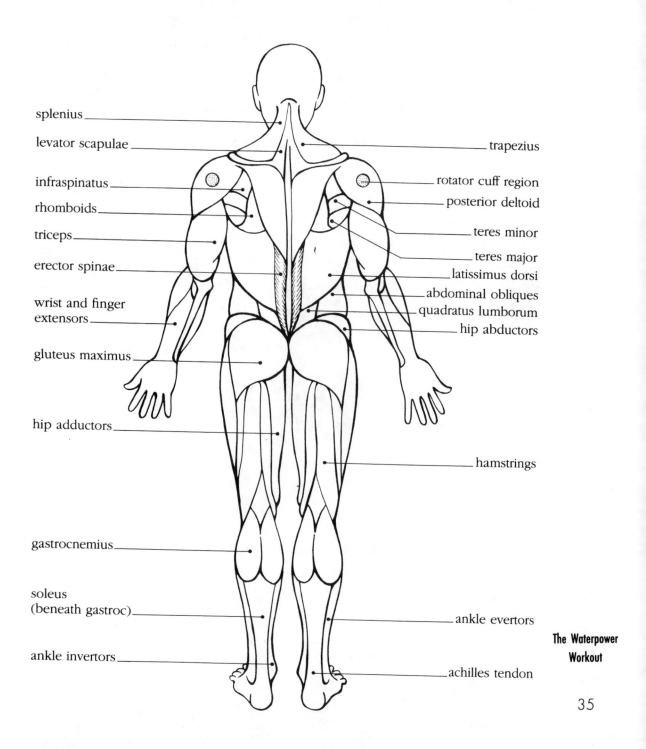

splenius

levator scapulae

infraspinatus

rhomboids

triceps

erector spinae

wrist and finger
extensors

gluteus maximus

hip adductors

gastrocnemius

soleus
(beneath gastroc)

ankle invertors

trapezius

rotator cuff region

posterior deltoid

teres minor

teres major

latissimus dorsi

abdominal obliques

quadratus lumborum

hip abductors

hamstrings

ankle evertors

achilles tendon

**The Waterpower
Workout**

35

Exercise 1. Lunges

*Quadriceps, hip flexors, gluteus maximus, hamstrings, deltoids,
pectorals, latissimus dorsi, hip adductors*

Bend your right knee and place your right foot a full stride ahead of your left foot. Your left arm should be forward for counterbalance (Photo 1). Jump up and switch arm and leg positions so that the left leg is now forward and the right arm is forward. Each right-left cycle should be counted as only one repetition. **This is the key *opposition* exercise, so make sure your right arm is forward with your left leg.**

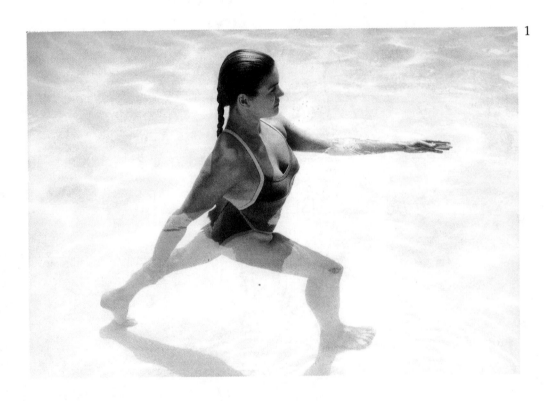

1

Exercise 2. Crossovers

Quads, hip adductors and abductors, pecs, deltoids, rhomboids, trapezius, triceps, gluteus maximus, hamstrings

Jump to a side-stride position with the legs slightly more than shoulder-width apart, the arms extended out to the sides at water level, palms facing out (Photo 2A). Jump again, crossing one arm and leg in front of the other, palms facing in (Photo 2B). Return to the starting position and alternate the arm and leg that cross in front on the return jump.

Exercises 3, 5, and 7 give a strong workout to the quadricep muscles, so a simpler recovery exercise is placed between them. Don't be surprised if you feel "quad burn." Even Olympic sprinters and jumpers experience this. Work through it while concentrating on form and rhythm.

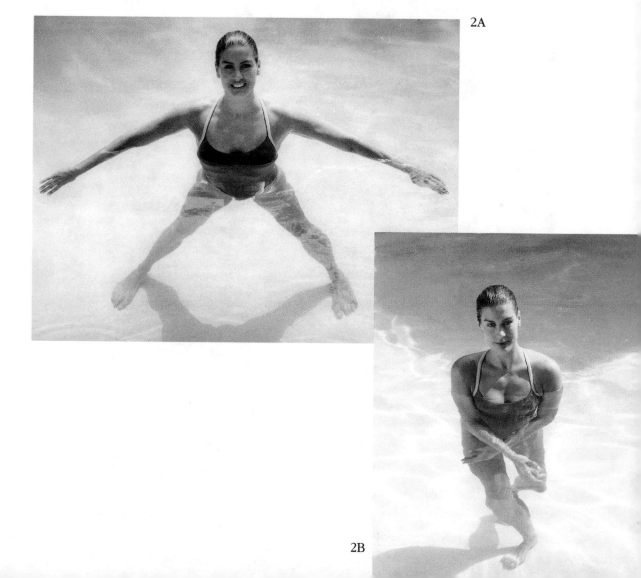

2A

2B

Exercise 3. Squat Jumps

Quads, hip adductors, gluteus maximus, hamstrings, hip abductors

Begin bouncing with your feet about shoulder width apart. Jump high and pull your legs together at the top of the jump (Photo 3A). Land with your feet apart (Photo 3B). Bend your knees as you come down and straighten them as you rise.

3A

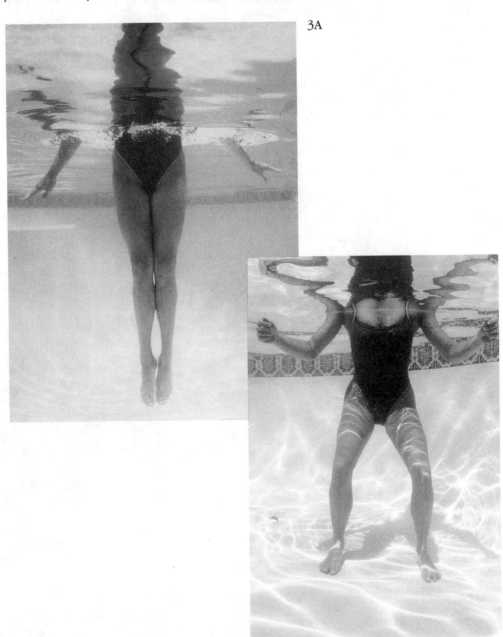

Exercise 4. Wide-Knee Running

Hip flexors, tensor fasciae latae, gluteus maximus, hamstrings,
quads, hip abductors and adductors

Hold your hands slightly below the surface of the water in a wide position. Lift your right knee to your right hand (Photo 4), then the left knee to the left hand. Every right-left cycle is one repetition.

4

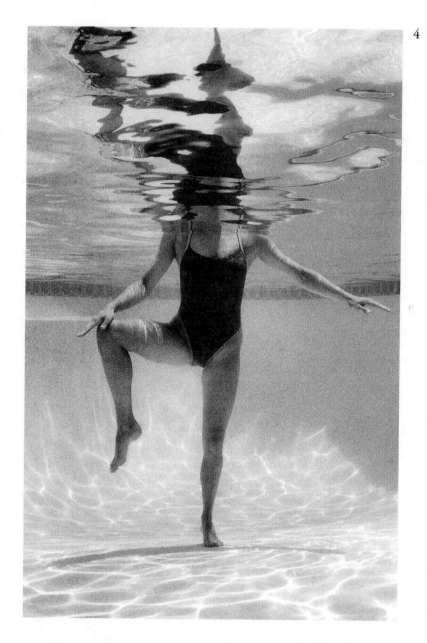

Exercise 5. Side-Straddle Jumps
Quads, hip adductors and abductors, gluteus maximus, hamstrings

Skip this exercise if you have a lower back problem.

Begin bouncing with the legs together. Jump up, open your legs wide apart (Photo 5), then pull them back together before landing on the pool bottom. Bend your knees as you land to regain your balance before the next immediate jump. Don't take extra bounces between straddles.

5

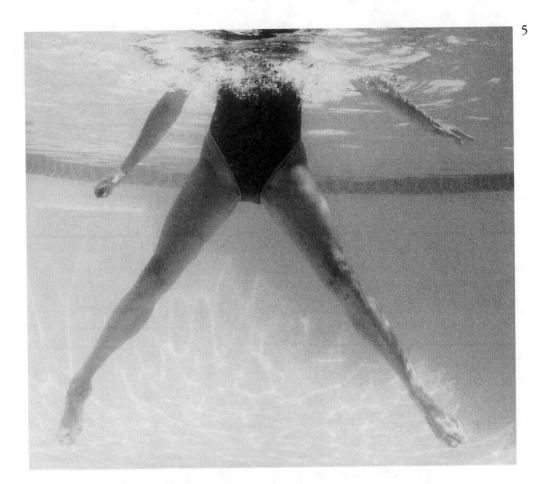

Exercise 6. Single Heel Lifts
Hamstrings, quads, gastrocnemius

Stand on your right leg and lift your left heel toward the buttocks (Photo 6). Lightly bounce, changing feet and snapping your right heel toward the buttocks. Keep your knees close together. Don't let your pelvis rotate back into a "sway" position. Use your abdominal muscles to stabilize the pelvis in a neutral position (see photos 6A and 6B, page 77). Add speed and strength until you feel the hamstrings working. Each right-left cycle counts as one rep.

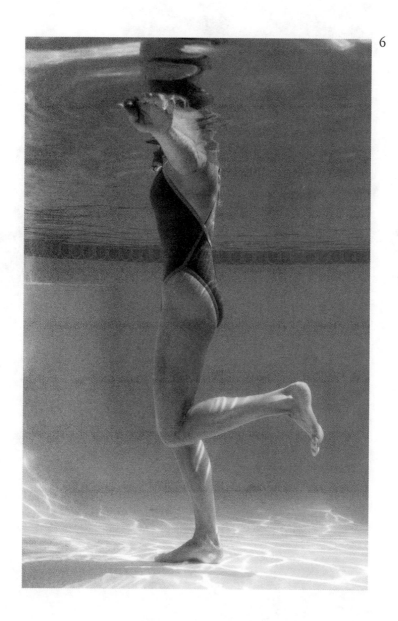

6

Exercise 7. Front-Straddle Jumps
Quads, hip flexors, gluteus maximus, hamstrings, hip adductors

Begin bouncing with the legs together. Jump up and swing the legs into a front split position (Photo 7A), then pull them back together before landing on the pool bottom (Photo 7B). Bend your knees for a soft landing and to allow extra time to regain balance before jumping up with the opposite leg forward in the split position. Each jump equals one repetition.

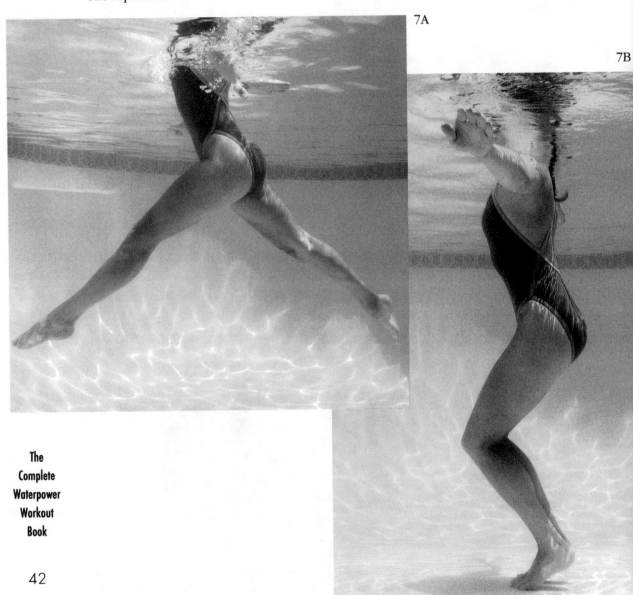

7A

7B

Exercise 8. V Kicks

Quads, hip flexors, hip adductors and abductors, abdominal obliques, hamstrings, gluteus maximus, pecs, lats, deltoids, teres

Stand on your right leg and extend your straight left leg up and out to the side at a 45-degree angle (Photo 8). Now bounce onto your left leg and lift your right leg up to the side, keeping it straight. Sweep both arms toward the leg that lifts. Swinging back and forth is one repetition.

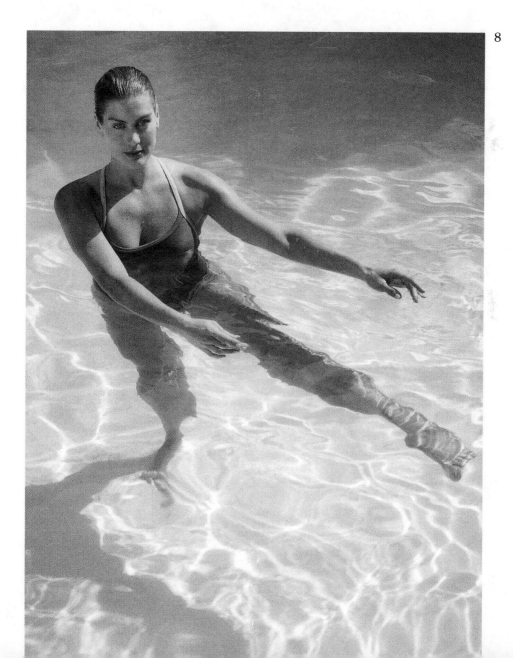

8

The Waterpower Workout

43

Exercise 9. Double Heel Lifts
Quads, hamstrings, gastrocnemius

Bounce with your feet pointing forward, comfortably apart. Jump high, keep your knees down, and powerfully lift both heels toward the buttocks (Photo 9). Concentrate on stabilizing your body with the abdominal and gluteal muscles. Land on both feet and immediately perform the next double heel lift.

9

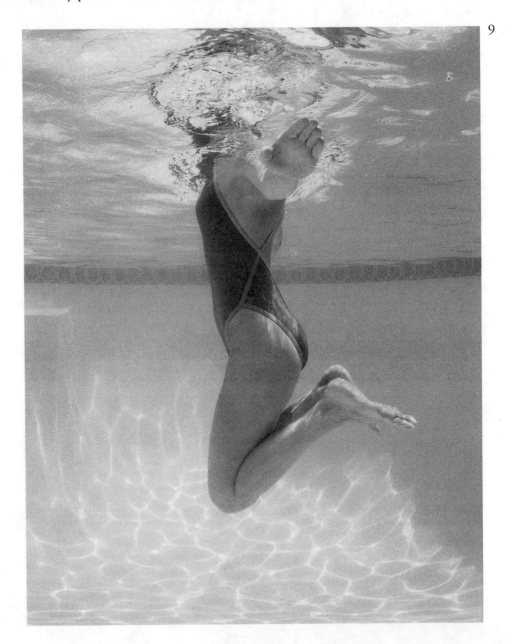

Exercise 10. Rocking Horse
Pecs, rhomboids, deltoids, trapezius, teres, quads, hamstrings, gluteus maximus, hip flexors

Bounce on your right foot and hold your left leg straight in front of you. Extend your arms straight out to your sides (Photo 10A). Rock forward onto your left foot and swing your right leg straight behind you. At the same time, sweep both arms through the water to position 10B. Now rock back onto your right leg, lifting the left leg straight in front and sweeping your arms back out to your sides. Continue rocking forward onto the left foot and backward onto the right foot, pulling your arms forward and backward with each rock. Push hard against the water in both directions. Palms face forward throughout the exercise. Perform half your reps like this, then reverse foot positions (right foot forward and left foot back) and perform an equal number of repetitions.

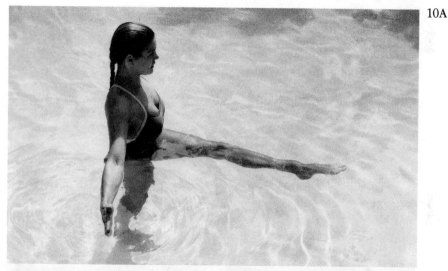

10A

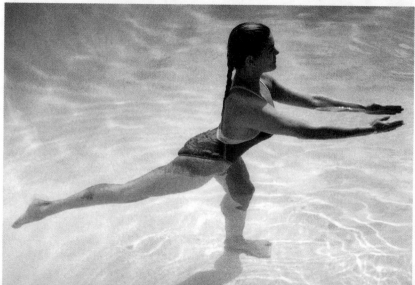

10B

The Waterpower Workout

Exercise 11. Leg Swings

Quads, hip flexors, gluteus maximus, hamstrings, hip adductors,
deltoids, pecs, lats

If you have lower back problems, shorten the movement of the swinging leg. Don't swing the working leg behind your body; just swing it in front, then down to the pool bottom (Photo 11A).

Bounce on your right leg with your left leg and right arm stretched out in front of you. Stay on your right leg as you swing the left leg backward with one bounce (Photo 11B), then forward with one bounce (Photo 11C). Your right arm swings forward and back at the same time as your left leg, your left arm swings opposite the right arm. Again, take the necessary time to make sure your legs and arms are moving in opposition. Perform half of your reps like this, then bounce on your left leg and swing your right leg for the other half of your reps. Do your best to keep the knee of the swinging leg straight throughout the exercise.

11A

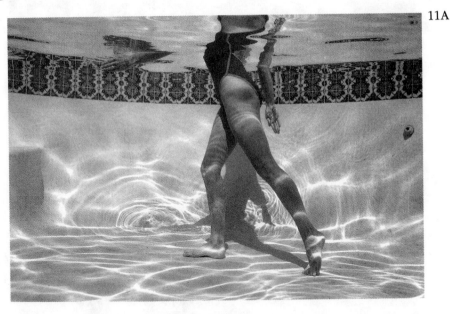

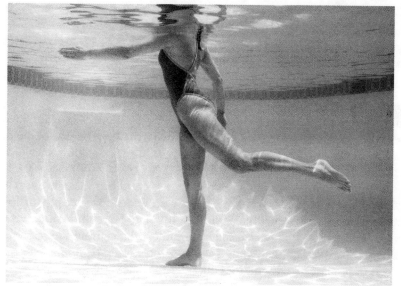

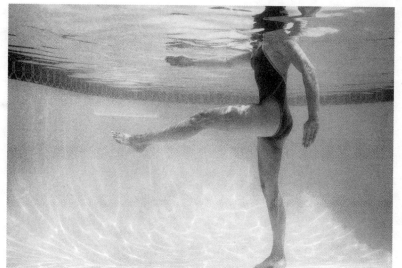

Exercise 12. Front Kicks

Quads, hip flexors, gluteus maximus, hamstrings,
hip adductors, lats, deltoids

The starting position for this exercise is the same as shown in Photo 11C. Lift your left leg straight out in front of you while you bounce on your right foot. Reach forward with your right arm for counterbalance. Jump up and switch arm and leg positions so that the right leg is now held straight in front of you and the left arm is forward. Each right-left cycle is one repetition.

Exercise 13. Back Kicks

Gluteus maximus, hamstrings, quads, hip flexors, erector spinae,
hip adductors, deltoids, pecs, lats

Skip this exercise is you have lower back problems.

Carefully assume the position in Photo 13 to work the gluteals forcefully while safely strengthening the back muscles. You can place both hands on the side of the pool while you learn this exercise. Then move away from the side and use your arms in opposition to the legs.

Stand on your right leg with your left leg straight behind you. Your left arm is forward, right back. Keep your chest forward and your chin down to protect your lower back. Jump and land on your left leg while swinging the right leg behind you and your right arm forward, left arm back. Squeeze the right gluteal throughout the movement. Now jump and land on your right leg while swinging the left leg behind, squeezing the left gluteal. Each right-left cycle is one repetition.

13

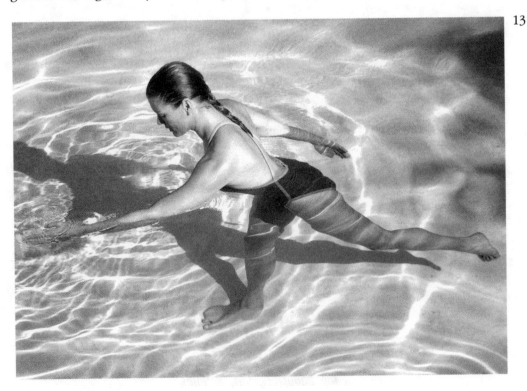

Exercise 14. Power Frog Jumps

Quads, hip flexors, gluteus maximus, hamstrings, pecs, biceps, triceps, deltoids, rhomboids, teres major

Bounce with your feet together and your arms stretched out to your sides at chest level. Jump off both feet and lift both knees toward your chest. At the same time sweep both arms forward to meet in front of you (Photo 14). Pull the arms back to their starting position as your feet return to the pool bottom.

14

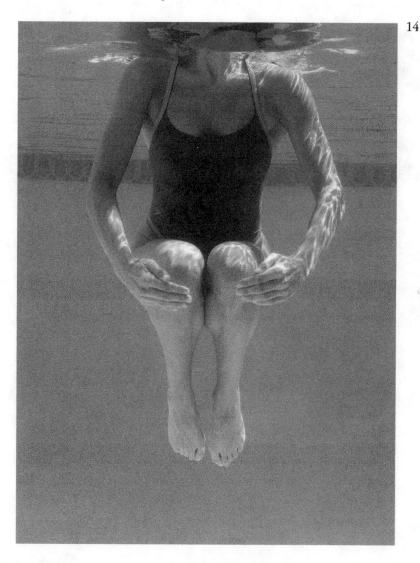

Exercise 15. One-Legged Frog Jumps
Quads, hip flexors, gluteus maximus, hamstrings, hip adductors, sartorius

Bounce on your right leg and hold your left knee bent in front of you as in Photo 15A. The left knee remains in this position throughout the exercise. Hold your arms anywhere out to your sides to help with balance. Now push off hard with your right leg and lift your right knee up to meet your left knee (Photo 15B). Then drop your right foot to the pool bottom. Bend your knee and prepare for another push-off. After finishing half your repetitions, change legs and perform the other half.

15A

15B

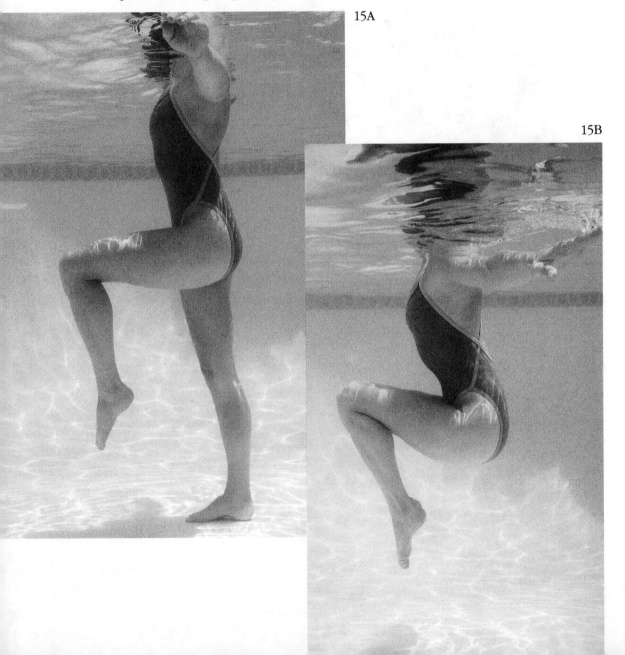

You are now ready for the anaerobic (see page 19) portion of your workout. You will be running in place and performing interval training. Monitor your heart rate throughout the interval training. (See box below.)

Working Heart Rate Target Zones

Women	Age	Minimum	Optimum	Maximum	Men	Age	Minimum	Optimum	Maximum
	25–29	130	157	185		25–29	137	166	195
	30–34	126	153	180		30–34	133	162	190
	35–39	123	149	175		35–39	130	157	185
	40–44	119	145	170		40–44	126	153	180
	45–49	116	140	165		45–49	123	149	175
	50–54	112	136	160		50–54	119	145	170
	55–59	109	132	155		55–59	116	140	165
	60–64	105	128	150		60–64	112	136	160
	65 +	102	123	145		65 +	109	132	155

Monitor Your Heart Rate

As you work harder during these intervals, your heart rate will increase. As you decrease the speed, your heart rate will slow. Thus, heart rate is the most accessible measurement of workout intensity. Although heart rate is usually spoken of in terms of beats per minute, you won't actually be monitoring your heart rate for an entire minute. Instead, you will count for six seconds, then add a zero—in effect, multiplying by ten. For example, if you count fifteen beats in six seconds, your working heart rate is 150 beats per minute. Because the heart rate begins to slow immediately upon ceasing exercise, you must begin this count without delay. The cooling effect of water seems to assist the heart in recovery, so the shorter pulse check is more accurate than a ten-second or fifteen-second count.

Scientific studies have shown that heart rates taken by manual palpation are often understated by as much as fourteen beats per minute. For more accurate heart-rate measurements, wireless, water-resistant **Polar Edge** and **Polar Accurex** heart-rate monitors should be used. A soft plastic strap with electrodes goes around the chest and a wristwatch displays the heart rate. The Polar Edge and Accurex pulse monitors let you see continuous digital heart-rate readings on the same screen as an elapsed-time stopwatch. Once you program the upper and lower reaches of your target heart-rate zone, the watch will beep if you fall below or work above that zone. After the workout, you can also read how long you worked in and above your target heart-rate zone.

Monitor your heart rate throughout the interval training with a Polar monitor or manually. See the chart above to determine your target heart rate. During exercises 1 through 15, your heart rate should fall in the low to middle portion of the target zone, but during intervals, your heart rate will climb to the highest end of the zone. If you go higher than appropriate for your age and sex, decrease the intensity (speed) of your interval training. If your heart rate is lower than your target zone, increase the speed of your running.

Exercise 16. Intervals
Biceps, quads, hamstrings, hip flexors, gluteus maximus, hip adductors, deltoids, pecs, lats

Begin running in place, simulating good form when running on land: The head and chest are erect, the shoulders are down and stable, eyes look straight ahead. The knees lift to 90 degrees while the arms pull directly forward and back—no lateral movement. Opposition is vital. Be sure the opposite arm and leg work together. There is no movement at the wrist or elbow, only at the shoulder. The angle of the arm at the elbow remains the same throughout the motion.

Once good running form has been established, begin increasing the pace. Try running at a slow, medium, and fast pace while maintaining good form. Then try sprinting in water (Photo 16A). If your form crumbles, begin again at a slow pace and work your way up to a sprint. Periodically monitor your heart rate (Photo 16B).

Now you are ready for intervals. A work period is followed by a slower recovery period, then another work period until you have completed five to ten minutes of intervals. You should continue jogging slowly during the recovery period. Do the appropriate sample workout:

A water-resistant Polar Accurex heart monitor offers the most accurate measurement of heart rate during intervals.

16A

16B

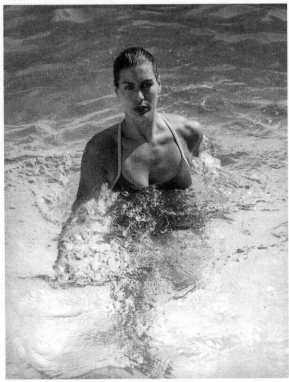

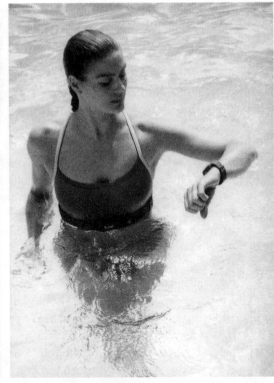

LEVEL 1

Thirty-second run
(heart-rate check)
Thirty-second recovery
Forty-five-second run
(heart-rate check)
Forty-five-second recovery
One-minute buildup (fifteen seconds each: slow, medium, fast, sprint)
(heart-rate check)
One-minute recovery
Forty-five-second run
(heart-rate check)
Forty-five-second recovery
Thirty-second run
(heart-rate check)
Thirty-second recovery

LEVEL 2

One-minute buildup (fifteen seconds each: slow, medium, fast, sprint)
(heart-rate check)
One-minute recovery
Three × thirty seconds (thirty seconds sprint, thirty seconds recovery, until three sprint reps completed, increasing speed on each sprint interval)
(heart-rate check)
One-minute recovery
Four × fifteen seconds (fifteen seconds sprint, fifteen seconds recovery, until four sprint reps completed, maintaining top sprint speed on all)
(heart-rate check)
Thirty-second recovery
Two-minute buildup, increasing speed every thirty seconds (thirty seconds slow, thirty seconds medium, thirty seconds fast, thirty seconds sprint)
(heart-rate check)
Move immediately to Exercise 17, Cool Down

LEVEL 3

Two-minute buildup, increasing speed every thirty seconds
>(heart-rate check)
>Thirty-second recovery

One-minute buildup, increasing speed every fifteen seconds
>(heart-rate check)
>Thirty-second recovery

Four × thirty seconds (thirty seconds sprint, thirty seconds recovery, until four sprint reps completed)
>(heart-rate check)
>One-minute recovery

Six × ten seconds (ten seconds sprint, twenty seconds recovery, until six all-out sprint reps completed)
>(heart-rate check)
>Move immediately to Exercise 17, Cool Down

Vary the length of your sprint intervals at each workout to keep this exercise fresh. For example, you may wish to run "step-ups" (fifteen, thirty, forty-five, sixty seconds) or "break-downs" (two minutes, one and a half minutes, one minute, thirty seconds) clocking equal work and rest periods. Or you may wish to run three to five intervals of the same length. If there's no clock at your pool, count arm strokes to measure the work bout, then recover until your breathing feels comfortable. To count arm strokes, count every time your right arm swings forward. A sample "arm stroke" workout might look like this:

>Twenty-five arm strokes easy
>Twenty-five arm strokes hard
>Recovery until breathing becomes easy
>Three × fifty arm strokes hard, with recovery between intervals
>One hundred arm strokes hard (Level 3 only)

Exercise 17. Cool Down
Quads, hamstrings, gluteus maximus, hip flexors, hip adductors

Run slowly from one side of the pool to the other and back in chest-deep water. Feel your rapid heart rate and breathing gradually subside. After two laps, change from a run to a two-footed jump. Continue crossing the pool, and after every lap (in a big pool) or two laps (in a small pool), change to the next:

- Two-footed jumps forward
- Two-footed jumps backward
- Right foot jumps forward
- Left foot jumps forward
- Right foot jumps backward
- Left foot jumps backward
- Bounding (Exercise 16, page 52)
- Backward running

Exercise 18. Back Flutter Kick
Hamstrings, quads, gluteus maximus, hip flexors, abdominals, hip adductors

Sit on a step or ledge, or turn your back to the wall of the pool and brace yourself with your arms on the gutter or edge of the pool. Lift your hips and legs and begin shallow kicking with straight legs. In all kicking exercises (18, 19, 20, 23, and 24), count one repetition each time your right foot breaks the surface of the water.

Exercise 19. Bicycling

Hamstrings, gluteus maximus, quads, hip flexors, hip adductors

Bend your knees and kick in a bicycling movement. For maximum benefit, lift the knee as close to the chest as possible, raise the foot out of the water, then pull the heel in close to the buttock at the end of each kick (Photo 19).

19

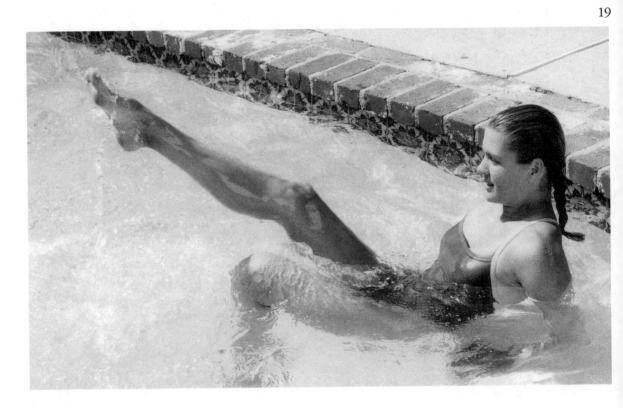

Exercise 20. Straight-Leg Deep Kick

Gluteus maximus, hip flexors, hip adductors, hamstrings, quads

If you have lower back pain, try this exercise slowly and with a narrow range of motion. If you don't experience any pain, proceed at a normal pace and gradually lift one leg higher and push the other one lower.

Straighten both knees as you lift your right leg to the water's surface and push the left leg toward the pool bottom (Photo 20). Moving with strength, change leg positions so the right leg sweeps toward the pool bottom and the left leg reaches toward the surface.

20

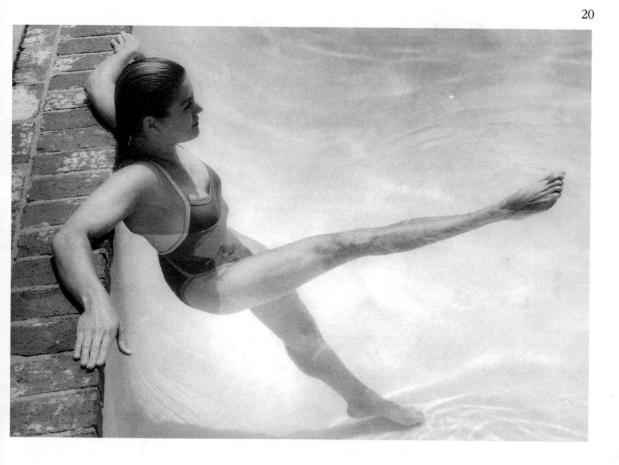

The Waterpower
Workout

Exercise 21. Scissors

Hip abductors and adductors, abdominals, quads, hip flexors, lats

Take the position in Photo 21A letting your lower back rest against the pool wall. Extend both legs straight out in front of you and open them to the sides. With a scissors motion, cross one leg over the top of the other (Photo 21B). Open them, then continue crossing and opening them, alternating the top leg. Use as much force in opening the legs as you use in closing them.

21A

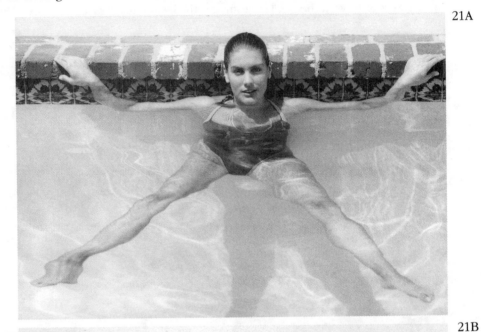

21B

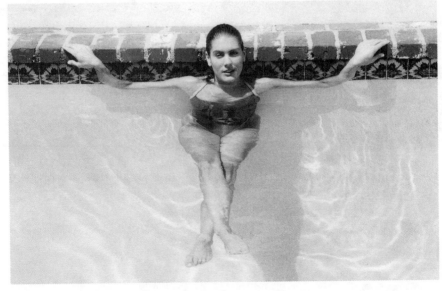

Exercise 22. Pendulum

Abdominal obliques, hip flexors, lats, hip adductors and abductors, quads

Stay braced against the pool wall as in the previous exercise, and hold both legs together straight in front of you. **If this hurts your lower back, bend your knees.** Keep your eyes focused straight ahead and don't move your head or upper body. Swing both legs as far as you can to the right (Photo 22), then to the left. Your contact with the pool wall will rock from one hip to the other. Each sideways swing counts as one rep.

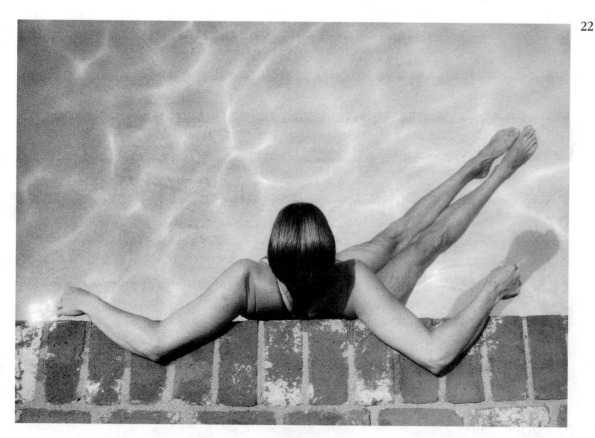

22

Exercise 23. Front Flutter Kick
Quads, gluteus maximus, hamstrings, hip flexors

Turn around and brace yourself facing the side of the pool. The hand position is the same as that in Photo 24. Hold the pool lip or gutter with one hand and place the other hand a foot lower to provide maximum leverage for maintaining this position. Lowering one hand also takes pressure off your lower back. Lift your hips and legs behind you and begin kicking with straight legs.

Exercise 24. Slap Kick
Quads, hamstrings

Your body remains in the same position as in Exercise 23, but now bend your right knee so the heel lifts almost to the buttock (Photo 24). Then slap the top of your right foot against the surface of the water as your left heel lifts toward the buttock. Continue, counting each right-left cycle as one repetition.

24

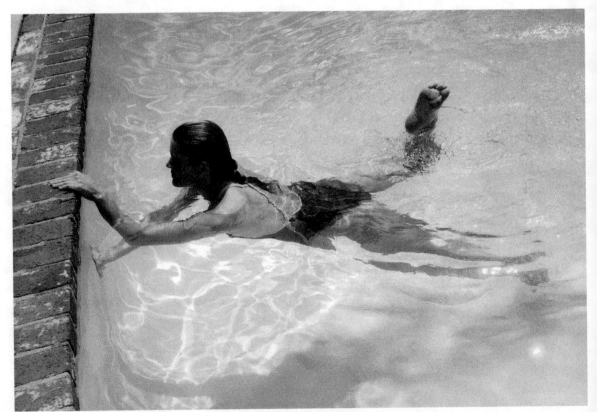

Exercise 25. Dips

Triceps, pecs, deltoids, lats, wrist flexors

If your pool has a gutter or railing, grasp it with fingers facing forward. If not, place your hands palms down on the deck in the most comfortable position you can establish. Now jump up and straighten your elbows, supporting yourself as in Photo 25A. From this position, lower yourself until the elbows have reached a 90-degree bend (25B). Then push back up to the starting position.

If this exercise is too difficult for you, be content for several weeks with holding yourself steadily in the starting position. Over the coming weeks you will be able to dip yourself to the low position. Begin with several reps, then gradually increase the number.

25A

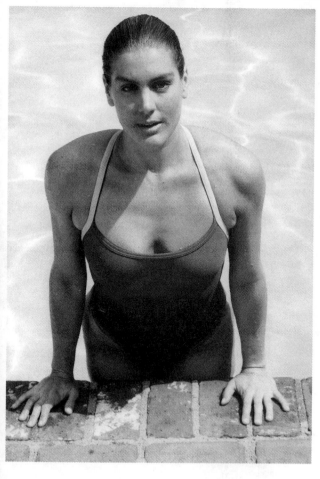

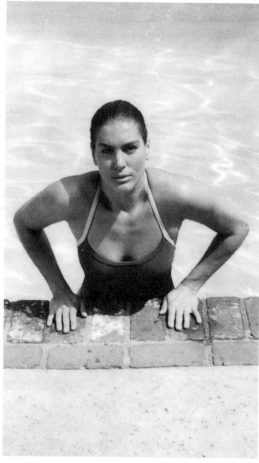

Exercise 26. Front/Back Pull

Pecs, trapezius, rhomboids, deltoids, infraspinatus, teres

Bend your knees until water covers your shoulders. Extend both arms straight out to your sides with your hands flat, fingers together, and palms facing forward (Photo 26A). Sweep your arms through the water to a clap in front of your body (Photo 26B). Maintaining the same hand position, pull your arms back to the starting position. Use equal force in both directions of movement through the water.

26A

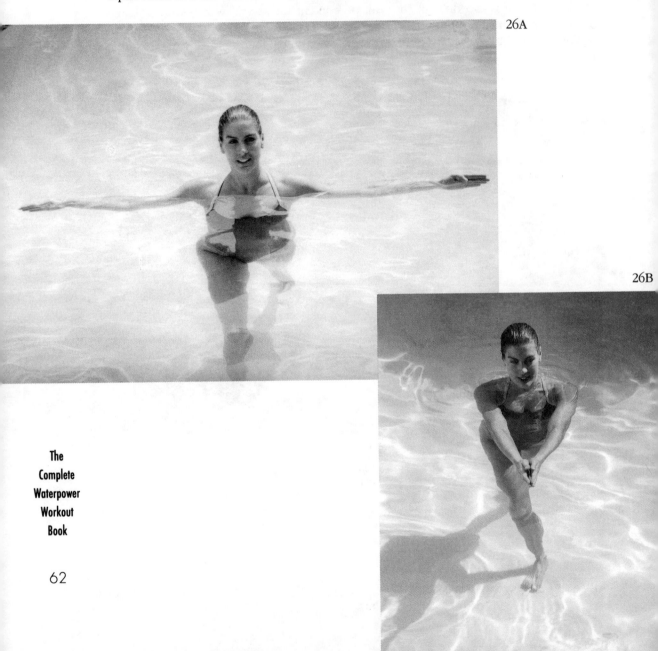

26B

Exercise 27. Up/Down Pull

Pecs, lats, trapezius, deltoids, teres, supraspinatus, rhomboids

Extend both arms straight out to your sides at shoulder level, palms down (Photo 27A). Hands are flat with the fingers held firmly together. Pull the arms down until your hands clap in front of your hips (Photo 27B). Without changing your hand position, lift the arms straight back to the starting position. Use equal force as you pull down and lift up.

27A

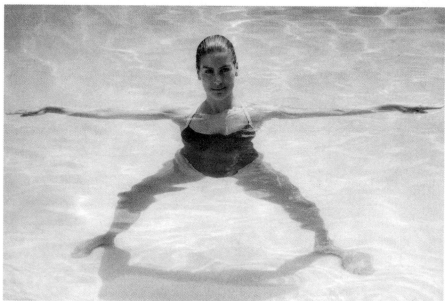

27B

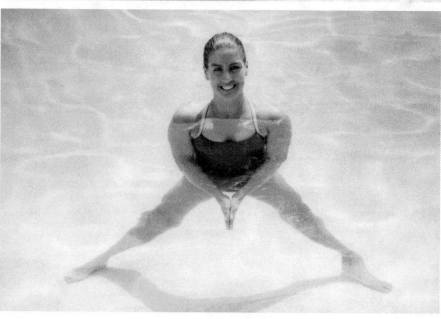

Exercise 28. Dig Deep

Lats, pecs, deltoids, teres, biceps, trapezius, triceps

Reach your arms straight out in front of your body, hands cupped and facing down (Photo 28A). Now pull your arms down past your hips as far behind your body as you can. Flip your palms to face forward (Photo 28B) and pull the arms forward until your cupped hands break the surface of the water in front of you. Flip your palms to face down again and continue. Each backward and forward pull is one rep.

28A

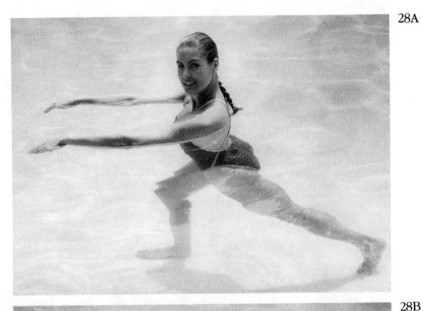

28B

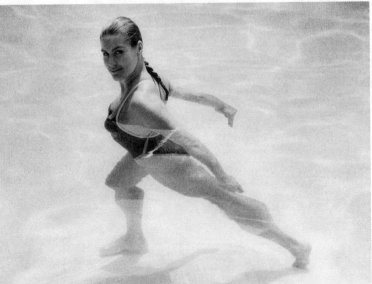

Exercise 29. Arm Curls

Biceps, triceps, wrist flexors and extensors

Touch the palms of your hands to your chest with your elbows wide and at the surface (Photo 29A). Hands are flat, fingers held firmly together. Hold your shoulders, elbows, and wrists stationary as you extend your arms straight out to your sides (Photo 29B). Only the lower arms move. Your elbows should not move forward and back, but should remain straight out to the side. If this is difficult for you, lean against the pool wall and keep your elbows in contact with the side as you swing the hands in and out. Use equal force pulling in and pushing out.

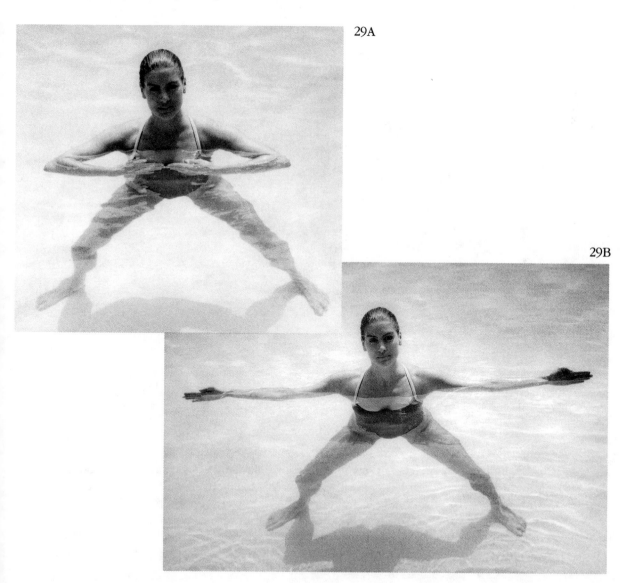

29A

29B

Exercise 30. Triangle
Lats, quadratus lumborum, hip abductors, abdominal obliques, teres

Stand with your feet wider than shoulder width apart. Lift your left arm straight up and over your head, letting your right hand slide down your right leg under the water (Photo 30). The hips face forward throughout this stretch. Do not twist to the side or bend forward from the waist. Allow the neck to relax by letting the right side of your head hang toward the water. Breathe slowly and deeply as you feel this exercise stretch the muscles of the left hip, arm, and shoulder. Repeat with the right arm.

30

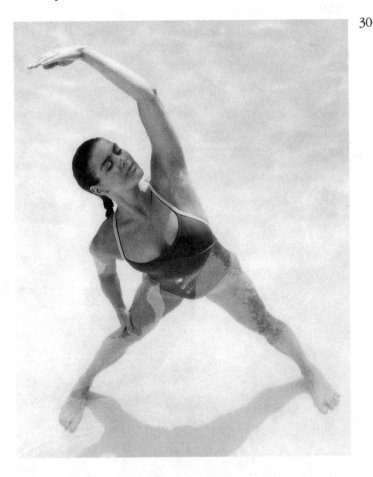

Beginning with Exercise 31, stand with your right hand on the side of the pool and your hips perpendicular to the pool wall. (Photo 31A). Perform half of your repetitions with the left leg and continue working the left leg through Exercise 35. Then turn around, place your left hand on the side of the pool and perform the second half of your repetitions for exercises 31 through 35, this time working the right leg. When performing exercises 31 and 32, do not lean your upper body to gain added leg height. Hold your torso steady even if the leg lifts only a short way.

Exercise 31. Lateral Leg Lifts

Hip abductors and adductors, glutals

Stand with your right hand on the side of the pool and your hips perpendicular to the pool wall. (Photo 31A) Maintaining erect posture, lift your left leg directly to the side (Photo 31B). Keep the feet parallel so that the knee points forward rather than upward. Lift the leg only as high as you can without altering your upper body position. Then pull your left leg back to the starting position.

Apply equal force as you lift the leg up and pull it down.

31A

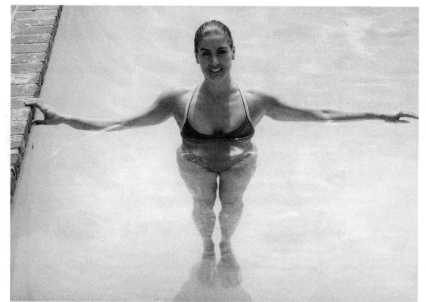

31B

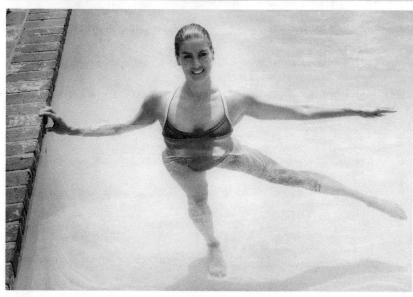

**The Waterpower
Workout**

Exercise 32. Leg Circles

Hip abductors and adductors, abdominals, gluteals

If you have lower back pain, skip this exercise.

Lift your left leg straight forward in front of you (Photo 32A), then smoothly continue the motion in a circle by swinging the leg out to your left side (Photo 32B), then behind you (Photo 32C). Complete the circle by brushing the left leg past your right leg, then beginning the next large circle. Reach as far as you can in each direction. Do half of your reps like this, then, without altering your body position, reverse the direction of the circle and perform the other half. Reach your leg behind you, then to the side, then the front.

32A

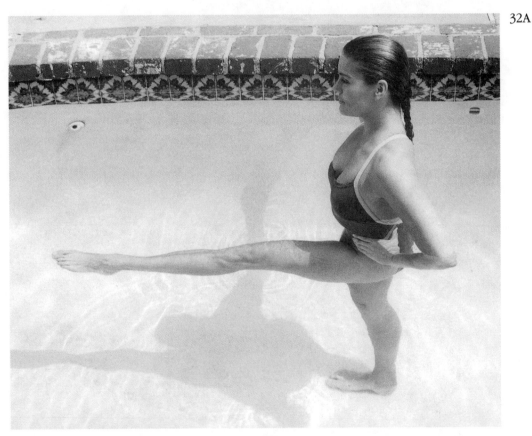

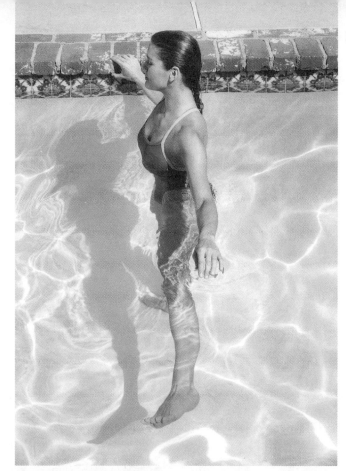

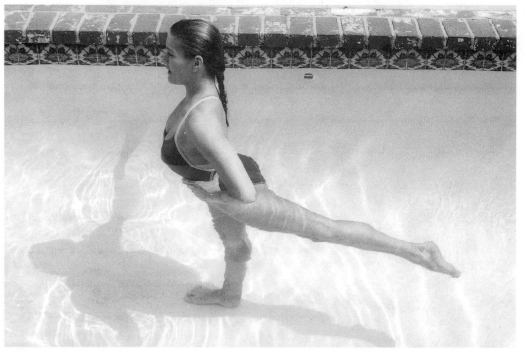

**The Waterpower
Workout**

69

Exercise 33. Knee Swivels
Hip flexors, hip rotators, hip abductors and adductors, sartorius

Skip this exercise if you have had hip-replacement surgery.

    Bend your left knee and lift it to be parallel with, but below, the surface of the water. Keeping the upper body stationary, swivel the knee out to the side as far as you can reach (Photo 33A), then cross it in front of the body (Photo 33B).

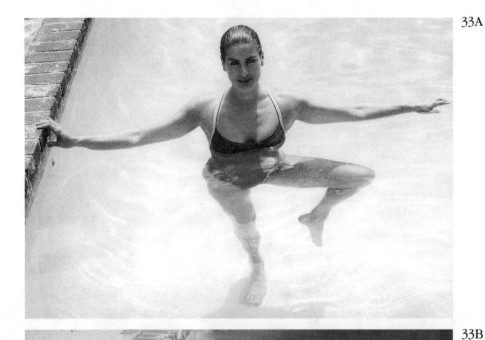

33A

33B

Exercise 34. Quad Extensions
Quads, hamstrings, hip flexors

Hold your left knee straight in front of you, foot dangling toward the pool bottom (Photo 34A). Kick the lower leg away (Photo 34B), then pull it back to the starting position. If this position causes back pain or is too difficult for you, lower the knee partway and kick from that position.

34A

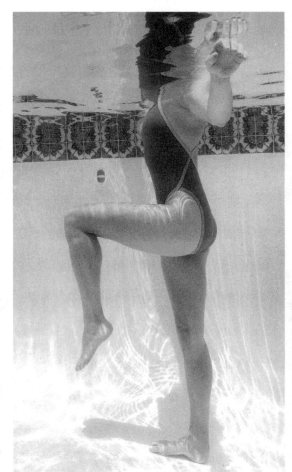

34B

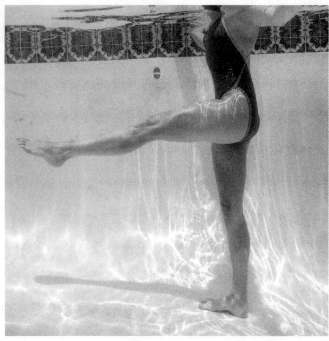

Exercise 35. Hamstring Curls
Hamstrings, quads, gastrocnemius

Start with your knees together, feet together on the bottom of the pool. Keep your knees together as you raise your left heel up toward the left buttock (Photo 35), then push your foot back to the starting position. Kick up and down with equal force, reaching for full flexion (bending) and extension (straightening).

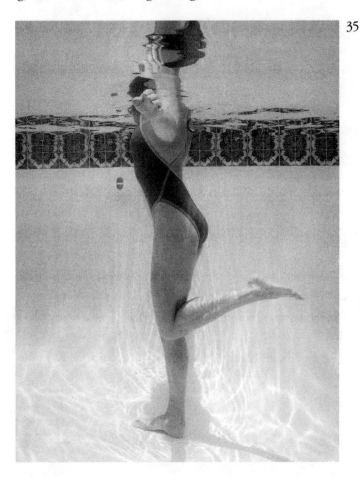

35

Now turn and place your left hand on the side of the pool. Repeat exercises 31 through 35, working the right leg.

Stretching exercises 36, 37, and 38 are to be done gently. Never force a stretch if there is pain. Stretch only to the point of discomfort, ease back a bit, then hold the position until the muscles have relaxed and lengthened. If you continue to feel discomfort, don't try harder. Relax more. If you tend to become chilled at this point of the workout, you can add a Wet Wrap for warmth as in Photo 37. (See also pages 8 and 9.)

Exercise 36. Quad Stretch
Quads

Stand facing the side of the pool, your right hand on the deck for balance. Bend your left knee and reach behind to grasp your left ankle with your left hand. Using your abdominal muscles, stabilize the pelvis into a "neutral" position to prevent "swaying." (See photos A and B, page 77.) Now pull the left heel up toward the left buttock and maintain steady pressure as you feel a stretch in the quadriceps muscles (Photo 36). Breathe slowly and deeply five to ten times. Place your left hand on the deck for balance and repeat with the right leg.

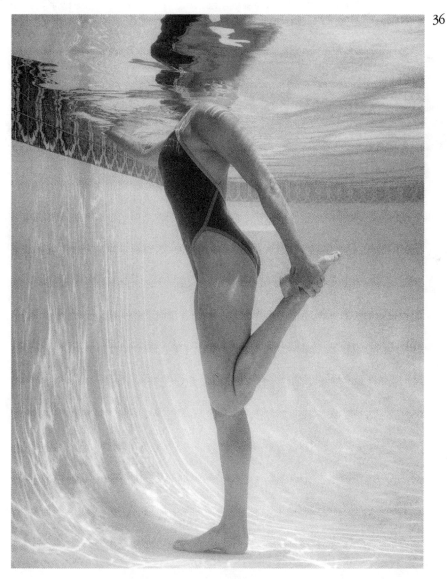

36

The Waterpower Workout

Exercise 37. Hamstring Stretch

Hamstrings, gluteals, gastrocs, erector spinae, rhomboids, trapezius

Face the side of the pool, and place your hands on the deck for balance. Lift your right foot straight in front of you onto the side wall of the pool. If you are quite flexible, your foot will approach the surface of the water. If not, your foot will be placed approximately knee height on the side of the pool. Place your foot where you feel a challenging stretch, but no sharp pain. Relax your shoulders, arms, neck, and back. Breathing slowly and gently, try to straighten your knee and push your heel toward the pool wall (Photo 37). If you experience any discomfort in your lower back, bend the knee and lower your foot. If your flexibility permits, try to rest your chest on your thigh, knee, or shin. Breathe slowly and deeply five to ten times. Repeat with the left leg.

37

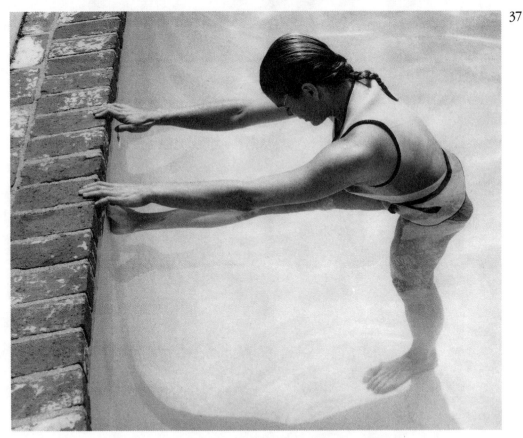

If you tend to chill at the end of the workout as you stretch, wear a Wet Wrap.

Exercise 38. Body Swing

Hip adductors, hamstrings, hip rotators, gastroc/soleus complex,
lats, biceps, triceps, quads

Get a good grip on a gutter, ladder, skimmer box, Hol-Tite restrainers, or the lip of the pool. Walk both feet up the pool wall to the position in Photo 38A. Now bend your right knee as far as you can and swing your body to the right, fully straightening the left knee (Photo 38B). Swing back to the left by straightening your right knee and fully bending your left. Swing back and forth several times, taking time to enjoy this pleasurable stretch.

38A

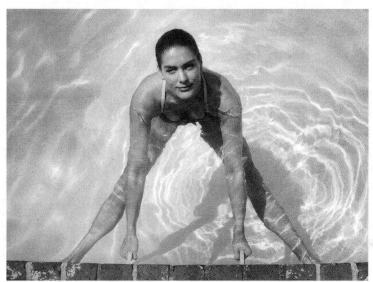

38B

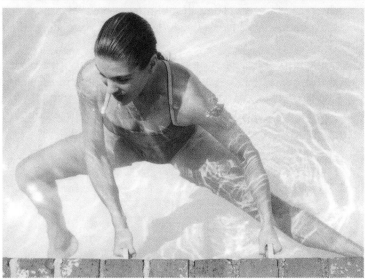

Time Out for Correct Biomechanics

Whether you sit, stand, walk, run, or perform any sports skill, there is a position, posture, stance, or alignment that helps the body perform the activity most smoothly, with the least effort or strain. When you use correct biomechanics, good form, your movements are more efficient. Most coaches and movement experts agree that good form is the primary building block of any activity. If you focus on only one thing while training, it should be good form. Then, once good form is established, you add speed.

For instance, if running in water seems difficult to you at first, slow down the speed and emphasize erect posture, level head position, arms driving straight forward, knees lifting to 90 degrees. Gradually increase the speed of the running *only* if you are able to hold form. Never work faster than your form will allow. If your form crumbles at any point, slow down and put the building blocks together again from the beginning.

Here are some general rules of correct biomechanics:

1. Imagine a string attached to the top of your head lifting it straight up to the sky or ceiling.

2. Keep your chest lifted toward the sky, but keep your shoulders relaxed and down.

3. Keep the head level, eyes focused straight forward. If the chin tilts up, the back arches and the hips sway back. If the chin tilts down, the body tends to curl inward.

4. Prevent rotational movements of the spine unless specifically asked to do them. Unnecessary rotation of the spine is an example of poor biomechanics that waste energy and over months and years can cause microtrauma or pain.

5. Maintain a neutral pelvic position. The natural tendency for many people is to allow the buttocks to swing backward, forcing the pelvis into a "sway" position and placing undue pressure on the lower back. Keep the abdominal muscles taut, the knees slightly unlocked, and you'll hold your pelvis in the neutral, correct position. (See photos A and B.)

6. Notice the position of your feet. They should remain parallel, toes pointing forward through all movements unless, like a ballet dancer, you have a specific reason for a turned-out position.

7. Be aware of the goal of each exercise you perform and try to isolate the muscles involved; don't move other body parts to generate a "whipping" action for added strength. For example, when doing leg circles, many people swing their entire bodies in order to move the legs. Instead, use only the muscles surrounding the hip to do the work and you'll gain more strength exactly where you targeted it.

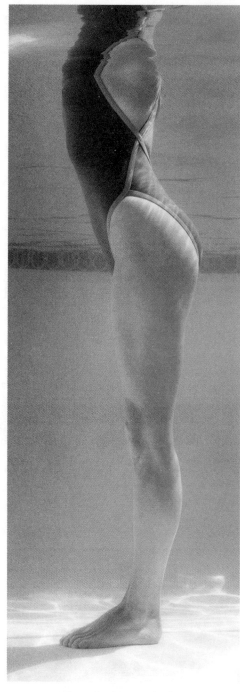

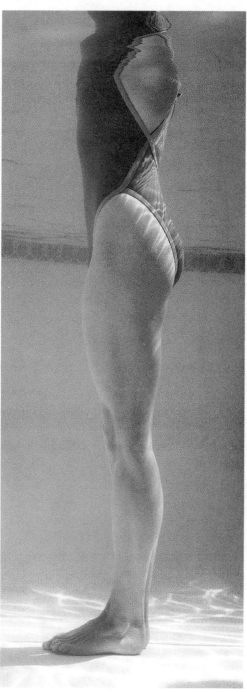

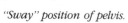

"Sway" position of pelvis.

Neutral position of pelvis

**The Waterpower
Workout**

77

The Twenty-five-Minute Powerhouse Workout

If time is short but you want an explosive, strenuous workout, do thirty repetitions of each of these exercises, in order, **with no recovery time between exercises:**

1. Lunges
2. Crossovers
3. Squat Jumps
4. Side-Straddle Jumps
5. Front-Straddle Jumps
6. V Kicks
7. Double Heel Lifts
8. Rocking Horse
9. Leg Swings
10. Front Kicks
11. Back Kicks
12. Power Frog Jumps
13. One-Legged Frog Jumps
14. Intervals (five to ten minutes)
15. Back Flutter Kick
16. Bicycling
17. Front Flutter Kick
18. Slap Kick
19. Quad Stretch (1 rep each side)
20. Hamstring Stretch (1 rep each side)

You'll leave the pool after only twenty-five minutes with your craving for a vigorous workout totally satisfied.

Circle these exercises on your photocopy of the summary sheets, or make a second copy and cut and paste these exercises onto one page. Laminate your new exercise chart and take it with you for a poolside review.

The Waterpower Workout

Level I: 14 reps *Level II: 20 reps* *Level III: 30 reps*

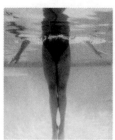

1. Lunges

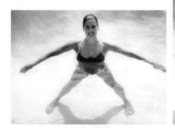 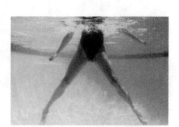

2. Crossovers
Alternate front arm and leg

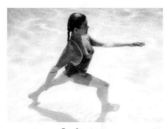 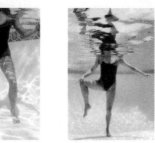 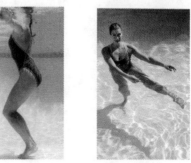

3. Squat jumps **4. Wide knee running** **5. Side straddle jumps**

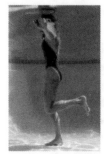 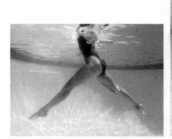 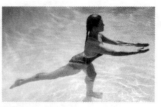

6. Single heel lifts **7. Front straddle jumps** **8. V kicks**
Alternate front leg

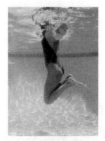 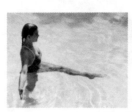

10. Rocking horse
Half reps with right foot forward
Half reps with left foot forward

9. Double heel lifts

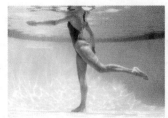
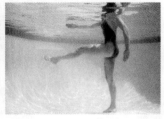

12. Front kicks

11. Leg swings
Swing right leg for half reps
Swing left leg for half reps

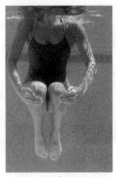
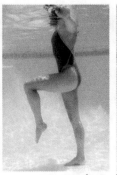
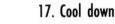
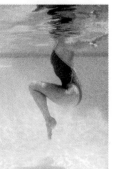

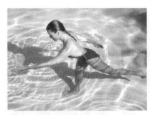

13. Back kicks   **14. Power frog jumps**   **15. One-legged frog jumps**
Half reps on right leg   *Half reps on left leg*

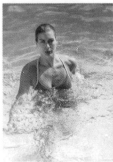

17. Cool down
Two-footed jumps forward
Two-footed jumps backward
Right foot jumps forward
Left foot jumps forwards
Right foot jumps backwards
Left foot jumps backwards
Bounding
Backward running

16. Intervals
Ten minutes of fast/slow running

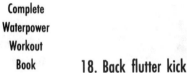

18. Back flutter kick

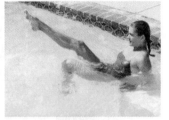
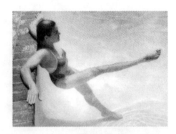

19. Bicycling   **20. Straight-leg deep kick**

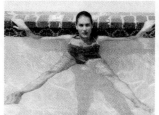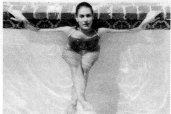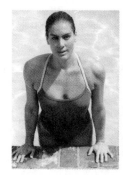

21. Scissors
Alternate top leg

22. Pendulum

23. Front flutter kick

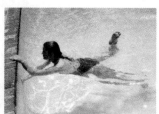

24. Slap kick

25. Dips

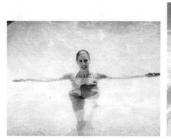

26. Front/back pull

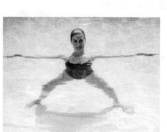

27. Up/down pull

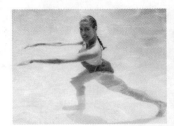 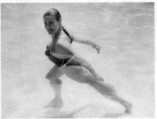

28. Dig deep

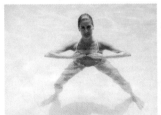 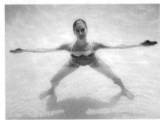

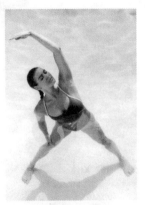

29. Arm curls

30. Triangle
One rep each side

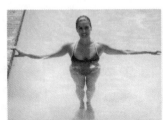 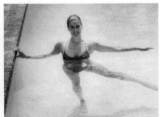

31. Lateral leg lifts

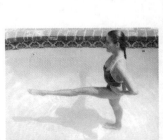 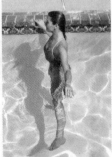 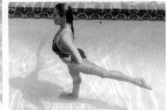

32. Leg circles
Half the reps in each direction

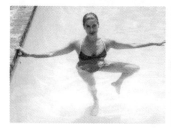
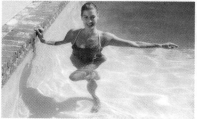

33. Knee swivel

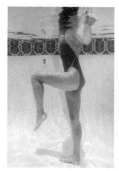
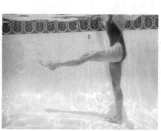
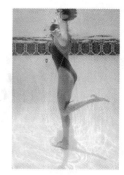

34. Quad extensions

35. Hamstring curls

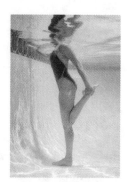
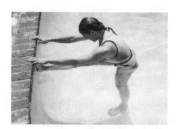

36. Quad stretch
One rep each side

37. Hamstring stretch
One rep each side

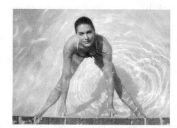
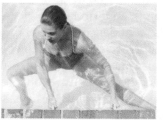

38. Body swing
Six to ten reps each side

The Waterpower
Workout

83

Three

The Deep
Waterpower Workout℠

A s with all water exercise, you can train as gently or as powerfully as you wish with
The Deep Waterpower Workout. If you are just beginning an exercise program, you
can move slowly and let your body gradually adjust to the new demands you are placing
on it. Then, as you become stronger, you can pick up the pace. The faster you move,
the more water resistance you encounter, and the harder your muscles have to work.
Remember: You don't need to know how to swim to exercise in deep water. Under the
close supervision of an instructor or lifeguard, your flotation devices will hold you up
and give you the confidence you need for even the swiftest water running. If you have
a fear of water, don't let that fear keep you away from the joy of water exercise. Many
hundreds of nonswimmers are now strapping on flotation devices and training gracefully in deep water that previously would have frightened them. **If you are a nonswimmer, do not enter deep water unless supervised and wearing the appropriate
flotation vest or belt.**

Because your feet don't touch the ground in these suspended maneuvers, it may take
a little longer to learn the exercises. Balance is the key. Once you learn where your center

of gravity is, you will be able to maintain and control your upright position. When you learn to use your arms and legs for counterbalance, you will be able to perform the various moves easily.

In virtually every deep-water exercise, the abdominals are the primary stabilizers for the body, so extra work on balance means additional work for the abdominals, which pays off in the development of a strong, defined abdomen.

The Deep Waterpower Workout uses interval training to provide you with a thorough aerobic and anaerobic workout. Other exercises strengthen the body's major muscle groups, and stretching exercises increase your flexibility. Since the feet don't push off the pool bottom, the calf and foot muscles don't work powerfully as they do in shallow water. So it is necessary to flex and point the toes on assorted exercises to add work for these muscles.

The cornerstone of any deep-water routine is water running and water walking. On land, running is a more strenuous activity than walking. The reverse is true in water because moving straight arms and straight legs through water's resistance is more difficult than moving limbs that are bent as in running. These key moves are described in detail in exercises 1 and 2. Dancers and runners usually conquer these skills in deep water right away; others may take much longer. If you experience some difficulty, and many people do, focus on developing opposition: Make sure your left arm moves in sync with your right leg and your right arm works in time with your left leg. (See page 11 for a fuller explanation.)

What Equipment Do I Need?

The first step in deep-water work is to select the flotation device that best holds you in a comfortable upright position for exercising. The Appendix gives you information on where to find the equipment listed below. Photos appear throughout this chapter.

The Wet Vest, Wet Vest II, and The Wet Belt. The Wet Vest was the first flotation device designed specifically for deep-water running. The Wet Vest II improves on the design to eliminate chafing around the arms and allow for a wider range of body sizes to use the same piece of equipment. Vests help keep you warm if you exercise year-round in an outdoor pool. The Wet Belt, which fits all waist sizes, is the easiest to put on of all flotation pieces because it straps on with a wide band of Velcro. It provides greater buoyancy even for athletes with a low percentage of body fat who don't float easily.

The AquaJogger. The AquaJogger was the first buoyancy belt manufactured for deep-water exercise. Its positioning eliminated the vest's chafing problem in the arm and crotch area. Like the flotation belts that were developed later, the AquaJogger allows for full range of motion of both arms and both legs in all body positions, from vertical to horizontal. The AquaJogger is held around the waist by an adjustable, elastic belt with a quick-release buckle. It is particularly well suited for those with lower back problems because its wide design provides stability and support for the lower back.

Aqua Belt. The Aqua Belt comes in two styles. The streamlined model is rectangular and fits snugly to the body with quick-release buckles and adjustable straps. Most other belts are more than one inch thick, which forces a slightly wide arm carriage in water running and water walking. The Aqua Belt Streamliner is only ¾ inch thick and thus allows more accurate arm movement. Athletes, dancers, or anyone below 15 percent body fat should consider the higher-buoyancy Aqua Belt Deluxe model, which is over one inch thick.

Wet Sweat. This teal-colored belt provides extra buoyancy for those with low body-fat percentages. Clasps are a combination of quick-release buckle and adjustable strap with Velcro to keep the loose end of the strap under control. The new color and shape make it popular with students.

Other flotation belts. Standard water-ski belts are a versatile, inexpensive option. They are a vital tool for swimmers with lower back pain. (See pages 255–260 for details.)

Hydro-Fit buoyancy cuffs and hand buoys. Buoyancy cuffs can be strapped around the upper arms, the ankles, or the waist. When positioned around the upper arms, they increase the confidence of nonswimmers. Around the ankles, buoyancy cuffs give deep-water runners a sensation closer to land running by demanding additional downward thrust from the legs. In the ankle position they require greater strength and balance from the participant and aren't recommended for nonswimmers. Hand buoys add stability and resistance to deep-water exercises. If you choose the Hydro-Fit buoyancy system of cuffs and buoys, eliminate exercises 9 and 12 from your Deep Waterpower program and remove your equipment for exercises 17 through 28.

In selecting the flotation device that is right for you, keep in mind whether or not you float easily. If you have a low percentage of body fat (under 15 percent), or if you know you are a "sinker," be sure to ask for extra buoyancy on your Wet Vest, Wet Vest II, or request the "EB" AquaJogger.

If your pool is small, or if you find turning back and forth during water running distracting to your workout, simply add a Waterpower Workout Tether or Perry Band around your waist. Now you can focus strictly on your speed as you run in place. You can even close your eyes if you wish.

The Waterpower Workout Tether. This device buckles like an old-fashioned airplane seat belt, and because it comes in sizes, will fit snugly around your waist. One end of the elasticized tether attaches to the buckle on your waistband. The other end attaches to a ladder, a railing, or your coach's ankle. The movable D-ring lets you position the elasticized tether precisely in the middle of your back.

The Perry Band. This waistband threads through a plastic buckle and folds back on itself with Velcro. The ankle strap attaches to a ladder, railing, or piece of lawn furniture. One size fits all, so if you have a small waist, don't try to tighten the waistband to fit snugly; you will pull it taut when you begin running.

Tips for Deep-Water Workouts

Once outfitted, slide into deep water and begin warming up with Exercise 1, Water Running. Keep these tips in mind:

- Take time to learn good form for both water running and water walking. They are the two most important components of your workout, and should be done correctly to maximize the benefits of the exercise. You may not notice that your arms are crossing the midline of your body as you run and therefore causing compensatory movements from your legs and spine. Or you may hang your head forward causing your shoulders to round, resulting in decreased breathing capacity and poor posture. Tips for correct form appear in exercises 1 and 2, but you may want to hire a coach for a session or two. It's easier to learn something correctly the first time than to break bad habits and have to relearn the movements properly later.

- **Begin all water-walking intervals slowly. A lot of force is required to swing straight legs through the water's resistance. It is possible to strain your hip flexors from working too rapidly too soon, so work up to top speed very gradually over several weeks time.**

- As you water run, you will move around the pool. Don't be surprised, however, if you stay in place during water walking. Many people do.

- Push and pull your arms through the water with equal power so you won't move around the pool during exercises 4 through 7, 10 through 12, and 15 through 17. If you find yourself moving forward or backward, you are pushing harder with your arms in one direction than the other. If you are turning left or right, one arm is working harder than the other. Concentrate on working both arms equally in both directions of the movement and you not only will stay in place, but you will also be strengthening your upper body more symmetrically. (See page 10 for a fuller explanation.)

> ## LEVEL 1

Follow the Level 1 program if you have not exercised for six months or longer, if you are pregnant, or if you're recovering from surgery, injury, or childbirth.

Sets and repetitions: One set of twenty reps of each exercise with a thirty-second rest interval between each exercise.

Frequency: Two to three days a week.

To progress: Add reps up to thirty, keeping a rest interval after each exercise. Progress to Level 2.

The Deep
Waterpower
Workout

Follow the Level 2 program if you have been participating in aerobic exercise regularly for two to three days a week for two months or longer.

Sets and repetitions: One set of thirty reps of each exercise. Add a fifteen-second rest between exercises *only* if you need it.

Frequency: Three to four days a week.

To progress: Add reps to forty, inserting fifteen-second or thirty-second rest intervals *only if needed* between exercises. Progress to Level 3.

LEVEL 3

Follow the Level 3 program if you have been participating regularly in aerobic and anaerobic activity three to four days a week for six months or longer.

Sets and repetitions: One set of forty reps with no rest intervals, then an extra set of Abdominals and Back Kicks.

Frequency: Four to six days a week.

To progress: When this level becomes comfortable, increase your speed during intervals or add Speedo SwimMitts to increase resistance.

The primary muscle movers are again listed in their order of importance.

As mentioned previously, the abdominal muscles of the stomach and erector spinae muscles of the back stabilize the torso in all deep-water exercises. These muscles will be listed only when they are acting as prime movers in the exercise.

Exercise 1. Water Running
Pecs, deltoids, biceps, lats, rhomboids, trapezius, hip flexors, hip adductors, gluteus maximus, hamstrings, quads

The
Complete
Waterpower
Workout
Book

88

Begin running in an upright position. Use the exact motion of good running form on land (Photo 1A). Your head and chest are erect; shoulders are relaxed and down. Eyes focus straight ahead to keep the head level. Knees lift to 90 degrees while the arms pull forward and back with no lateral movement. Hands are relaxed with relaxed thumbs facing up. Pull the elbows back, each in its turn, and touch each hand to an imaginary hip pocket.

Don't lean too far forward or you'll be dog paddling (Photo 1B). Simply lift the knee, then push the foot straight down behind you. Don't lean too far back or you'll have a tendency to kick forward into a bicycling motion (Photo 1C).

Jog for three to five minutes for a warm-up.

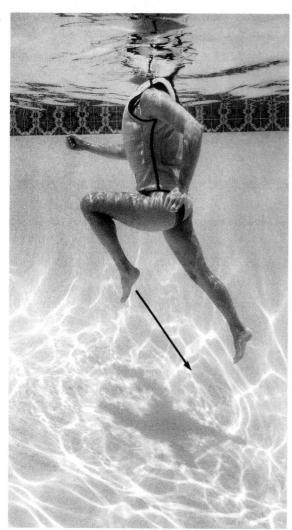

1A

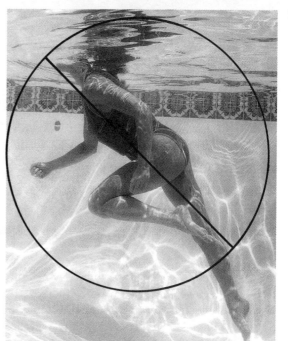

1B

Don't lean too far forward.

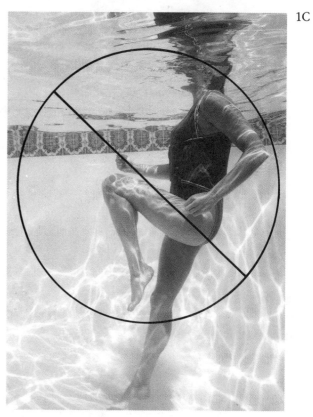

1C

Correct Water Running form. Foot pushes directly down and back, not bicycling forward as shown in Photo 1C. (Wet Vest pictured.)

Don't lean too far back.

Exercise 2. Water Walking

Hip flexors, gluteus maximus, deltoids, lats, pecs, hamstrings, quads,
hip adductors, trapezius, rhomboids, triceps
Power Walk only: Gastroc/soleus complex, tibialis anterior

Start by establishing an "opposition position." Hold your right arm forward and extend your left leg forward at the same time. Then begin walking, keeping both your arms and legs straight. Visually check your elbows and knees. Most people think these joints are straight when they are not. Stay upright; don't lean forward or back. If you lean forward, you won't see your legs in front of you at all. If you lean back, your legs are strictly in front of you. You should swing your arms and legs as far to the front of you as they swing to the back. In this way, the front and back of the body are worked equally. Water walk for one to two minutes or until you feel confident of the movement (Photo 2A).

Once the basic water-walking form becomes second nature to you, make it more difficult by turning your hands to a wide paddlelike position and adding lower leg work. (Photo 2B.) This is called the Power Walk position. Flex the foot of the leg that drives forward and point the foot of the leg that pushes back. This means that one foot is always flexing as the other is pointing. Use this Power Walk technique on the slow water-walking intervals and reach forward and backward as far as you can to work on flexibility. Turn your hands back to their original slicing position and eliminate feet movement during speed-walking intervals. Also during the speed walks, narrow the forward and backward range of motion of the legs so you can concentrate on greater speed. Focus on the backward pull of the leg and tighten the gluteal (buttocks) muscles on each backward thrust.

Having learned water running, speed walking, and power walking, you are now ready for your first set of intervals.

There are three sets in The Deep Waterpower Workout, broken up with deep-water exercises.

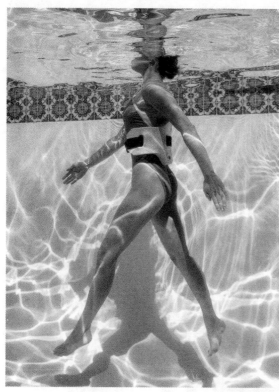

Basic Water Walking (AquaJogger shown)

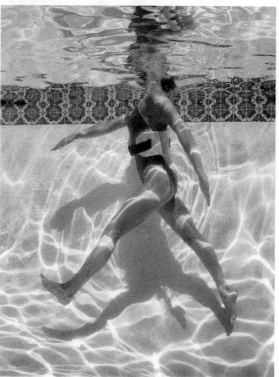

2B

Power Walk (AquaJogger shown)

The Deep Waterpower Workout

91

Exercise 3. Intervals—Set 1
See exercises 1 and 2 for muscle groups.

All these series of intervals start with low intensity and move to higher intensity. Be sure to monitor your heart rate where suggested. (See page 51.) In this way, you can either speed up to raise the heart rate or slow down to decrease the heart rate to stay within your target heart-rate zone. During recovery periods, power walk slowly, run slowly, or do flies (Exercise 10) slowly.

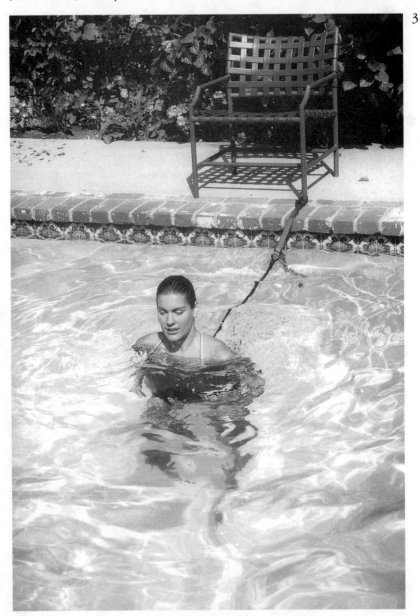

3

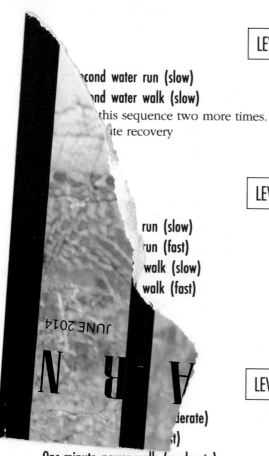

LEVEL 1

…cond water run (slow)
…nd water walk (slow)
  …this sequence two more times.
  …te recovery

One-minute water run (slow)
One-minute water walk (slow)
  (heart-rate check)
  One-minute recovery
  Repeat this sequence.

LEVEL 2

…run (slow)
…run (fast)
…walk (slow)
…walk (fast)

One-minute water run (slow)
One-minute water run (fast)
One-minute power walk (slow)
One-minute speed walk (fast)
  (heart-rate check)
  Repeat this sequence.
  One-minute recovery

LEVEL 3

…derate)
…t)
One-minute power walk (moderate)
One-minute speed walk (fast)
  (heart-rate check)
  Repeat this sequence.
  Thirty-second recovery

Thirty-second water run (moderate)
One-minute speed walk (fast)
  Repeat this sequence two more times.
  (heart-rate check)
  One-minute recovery

If you have been using a tether to stay in place for better concentration during these intervals, detach the tether now and move to an open space to perform deep-water exercises 4 through 8.

**The Deep
Waterpower
Workout**

Exercise 4. Bent-Knee Twist

Abdominal obliques, hip flexors, pecs, hip adductors and abductors,
gluteus maximus, deltoids, teres, biceps, triceps, hamstrings, quads, lats

Slightly bend both arms at the elbow while your feet dangle below. Lift your left knee across your body and meet the right elbow as in Photo 4. Repeat with the left knee meeting the right elbow. Each right-left sequence counts as one repetition.

4

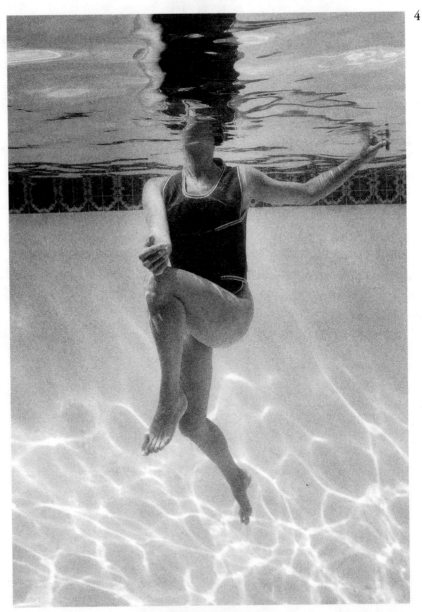

(Wet Vest II pictured)

Exercise 5. Straight-Leg Twist

Abdominal obliques, hip flexors, pecs, hip adductors and abductors,
gluteus maximus, hamstrings, quads, deltoids, teres, lats

Straighten your legs and continue the twisting movement as in Exercise 4, this time reaching not just for the right foot, but well past your right knee with your left hand (Photo 5). Repeat with the right hand reaching past the left knee. Each right-left sequence is one rep.

5

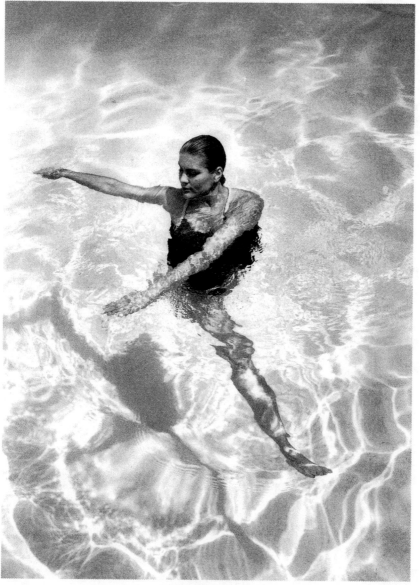

(Wet Belt pictured)

Exercise 6. Heel Lifts
Hamstrings, quads, gastrocnemius

Start from an erect position, your legs straight down toward the pool bottom (Photo 6A). Move your hands gently from side to side in front of you for balance. Keeping your knees pointed toward the pool bottom, lift both heels quickly toward your buttocks (Photo 6B). Then lower your feet toward the bottom of the pool, back to the starting position. The more snap you put into the heel lift, the more powerfully you contract your hamstrings. Do half of your reps lifting both heels simultaneously; do the other half of your reps kicking one heel up at a time. One snaps up as the other pushes down.

6A

6B

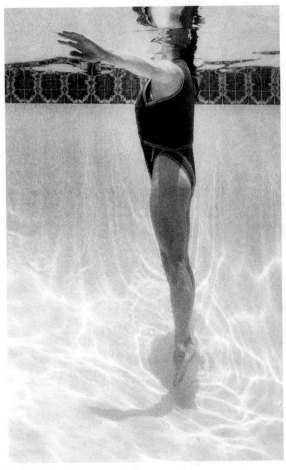

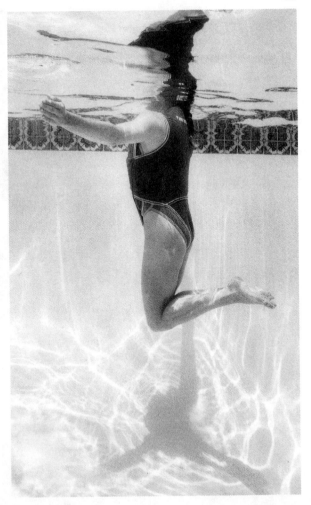

(Wet Vest II shown)

Exercise 7. Quick Scissors
Hip adductors and abductors, gluteus maximus, hip flexors

Continue sculling with your hands for balance, as your legs hang below you. Open your straight legs less than a foot apart (Photo 7A), then cross the right leg in front of the left (Photo 7B). Recross with the left leg in front. Emphasize quickness through a narrow range of motion. Each right-left crossing equals one rep.

7A

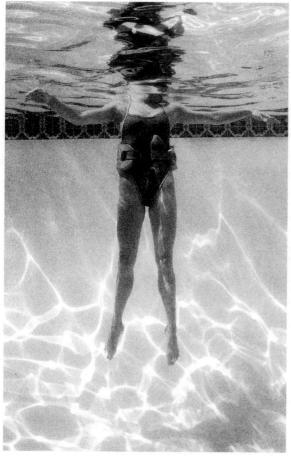

(AquaJogger shown)

7B

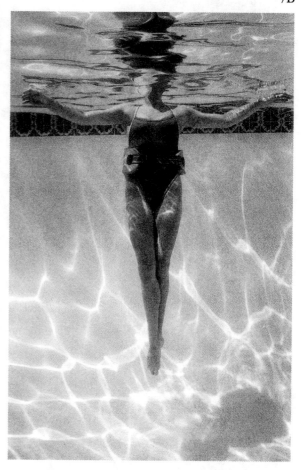

If you prefer doing your intervals on a tether, reattach yourself now for your second set.

Exercise 8. Intervals—Set 2
See exercises 1 and 2 for muscle groups.

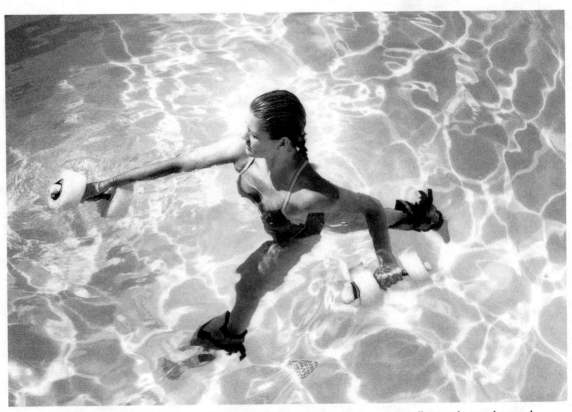

If you use Hydro-Fit buoyancy cuffs and hand buoys, perform basic water walking only, not the speed and power variations.

LEVEL 1

One-minute water run (slow)
One-minute water walk (slow)
   (heart-rate check)
   Repeat this sequence.
   One-minute recovery
Thirty-second water run (slow)

Thirty-second water run (moderate)
Thirty-second water walk (slow)
Thirty-second water walk (moderate)
   (heart-rate check)
   Repeat this sequence.
   One-minute recovery

LEVEL 2

One-minute water run (moderate)
One-minute speed walk (fast)
   (heart-rate check)
   Repeat this sequence.
   One-minute recovery
Two-minute water-run buildup, increasing pace every thirty seconds (thirty seconds each: slow, medium, fast, sprint)
   (heart-rate check)
   One-minute recovery
Two-minute water-walk buildup, increasing pace every thirty seconds (power walk during slow and medium segments; speed walk during fast and sprint segments)
   (heart-rate check)
   One-minute recovery

LEVEL 3

Three-minute water-run buildup, increasing pace every minute (one minute each: moderate, fast, sprint)
   (heart-rate check)
   One-minute recovery
Three-minute water-walk buildup, increasing pace every minute (power walk first minute; speed walk second and third minutes)
   (heart-rate check)
   One-minute recovery
One-minute water run (fast)
One-minute speed walk (fast)
   Repeat with no recovery
   One-minute recovery

**The Deep
Waterpower
Workout**

Exercise 9. Abdominals
Rectus abdominis, abdominal obliques, hip flexors, pecs, deltoids, trapezius, rhomboids, gluteals, triceps

Lean back to find a balance position in the water as in Photo 9A. Keep your legs together as you pull both knees toward your chest and your hands toward your knees (Photo 9B). Then turn your palms outward as you push your arms and legs back to the starting position.

Variation: Hold your arms gently to your sides and move them slightly if you must for balance. Lift both knees toward your right shoulder (Photo 9C), then return the legs to the starting position (9A). Next, lift both knees to your left shoulder, then extend the legs to the starting position. Continue alternating between right and left shoulders.

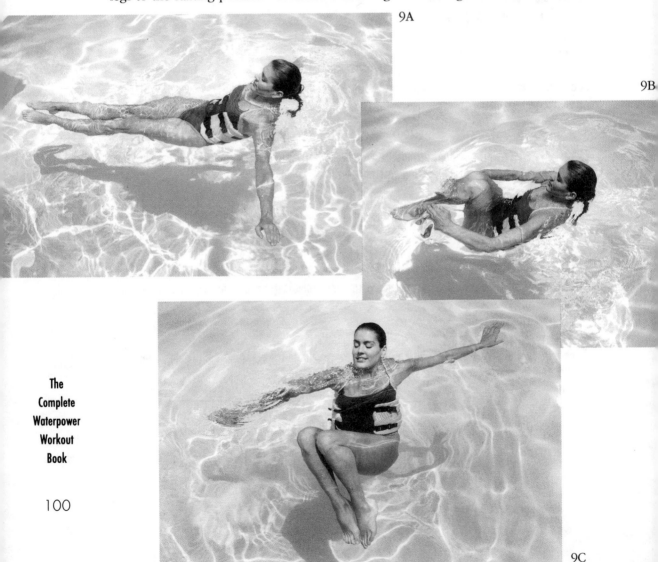

9A

9B

The
Complete
Waterpower
Workout
Book

100

9C

(Aqua Belt shown)

Exercise 10. Flies

Pecs, deltoids, teres, hip adductors and abductors, trapezius, rhomboids

Assume the position in Photo 10A: legs straight down and apart, arms straight out in front. Now pull the legs together as you swing your arms out to your sides (Photo 10B). Return with equal force to the starting position.

10A

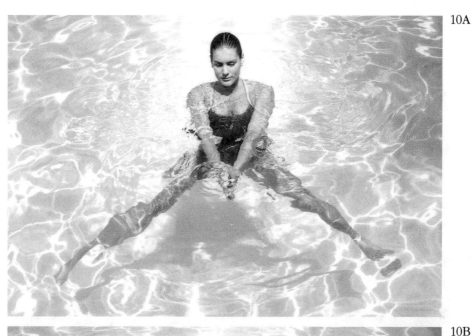

10B

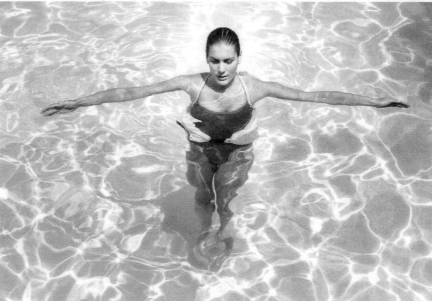

(Wet Sweat Belt shown)

Exercise 11. V Kicks

Hip flexors, abdominal obliques, tensor fasciae latae, pecs, deltoids, gluteals, hamstrings, teres, lats, trapezius, rhomboids

Swing your right leg up to a position right of center as in Photo 11. Under water both arms reach toward the right foot. As you next drop the right leg, lift the left leg to a position off center to your left, and swing both arms over toward the left leg. If you keep your arms straight and near the surface you will work your abdominals more than if you let your arms bend or drop low below the surface.

11

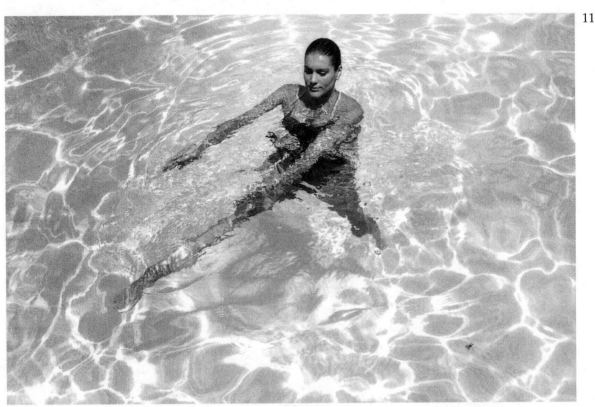

The
Complete
Waterpower
Workout
Book

102

Exercise 12. Back Kicks

Gluteus maximus, hamstrings, hip flexors

Skip this exercise if you have an acute lower back problem.

Carefully assume the position in Photo 12 to work the gluteals while safely strengthening the back muscles. Focus on moving *only* the legs; don't let your back arch with the leg swing.

Brace yourself on the side of the pool by grasping a ladder, skimmer box, railing, or lip of the pool deck with one hand and placing the other hand on the side of the pool below the water level, or use two Hol-Tite Restrainers. Lean forward and **look down at the water.** Let your hips float near the surface of the water as your left leg dangles below you. Lift your right leg straight back. Now switch leg positions. Once you learn the position and the movement, increase the speed to increase the work done by the gluteals. Each right-left sequence counts as one repetition.

12

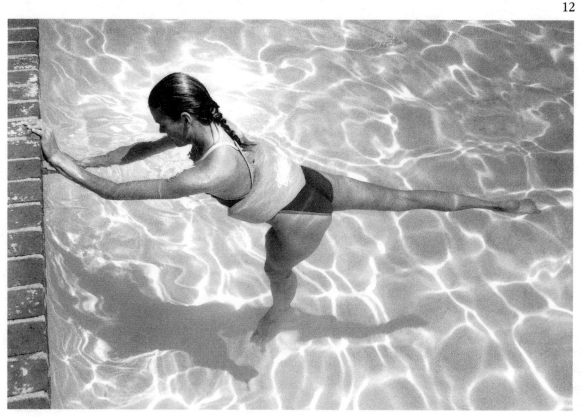

(Wet Sweat Belt shown)

Exercise 13. Intervals—Set 3

See exercises 1 and 2 for muscle groups.

Using what you've learned about interval training from the examples in exercises 3 and 8, create your own water-walking and water-running session that lasts five to eight minutes. Periodically monitor your heart rate to make sure you aren't working too fast or too slowly. Level 1 uses the basic water-walking technique. Levels 2 and 3 use the power-walking and speed-walking variations.

If you have access to shallow water, move to it now and remove your flotation device. If not, follow the directions below to help you maintain your balance while working your arms in deep water. The photos show the exercises being performed in shallow water.

Exercise 14. Up/Down Pull

Pecs, lats, deltoids, teres, supraspinatus, trapezius, rhomboids

Perform a gentle bicycling motion with your legs to balance you throughout this exercise. Extend your arms straight out to your sides at shoulder level, palms down (Photo 14A). Hands are flat with the fingers held tightly together. Now pull your arms down until your hands clap in front of your hips (Photo 14B). Without changing your hand position, lift your arms back up to the starting position. Use equal strength as you pull down and lift up. If this exercise brings your chin below water level, add more leg movement to counteract the powerful force of the arms.

14A

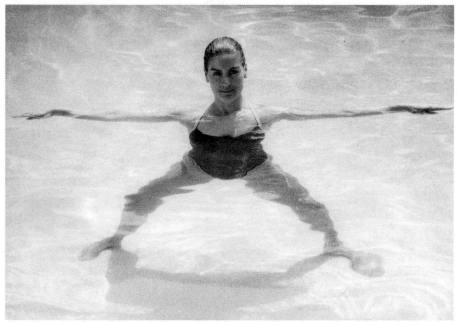

14B

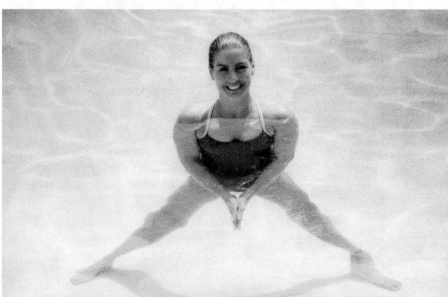

Exercise 15. Dig Deep
Pecs, teres, lats, deltoids, biceps, triceps, trapezius

Continue cycling for balance. Reach your arms straight out in front of your body, hands cupped and facing down (Photo 15A). Now pull your arms down past your hips and reach as far behind your body as you can. Flip your palms over (Photo 15B) and pull the arms forward until your cupped hands break the surface of the water in front of you.

15A

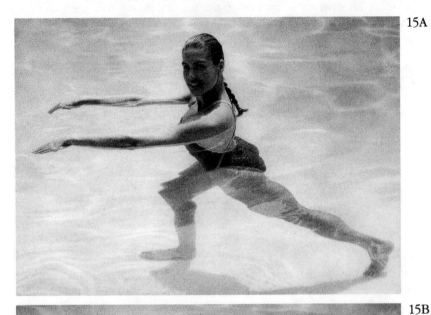

15B

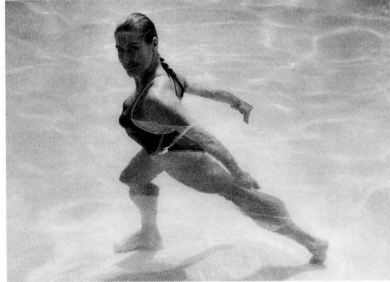

The
Complete
Waterpower
Workout
Book

106

Exercise 16. Arm Curls

Biceps, triceps, wrist flexors and extensors

Lean back slightly and continue cycling for balance. Touch your palms to your chest with your elbows wide and at the surface (Photo 16A). Hands are flat, fingers held firmly together. Hold your shoulders, elbows, and wrists stationary as you extend your arms straight out to your sides (Photo 16B). Only the lower arms move. Your elbows should not move forward and back, but rather remain straight out to the sides. Use equal force pulling in and pushing out.

16A

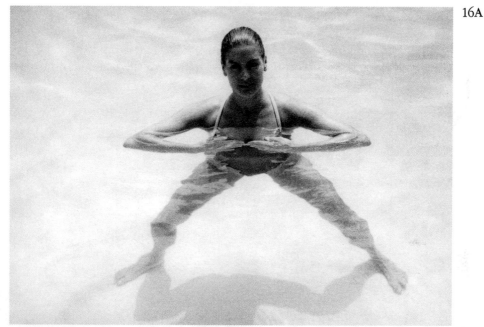

16B

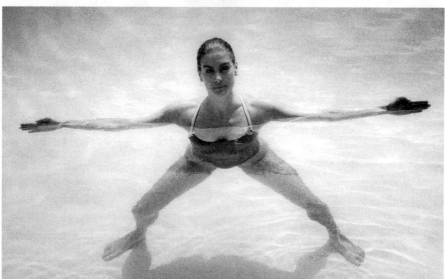

Exercise 17. Back Flutter Kick

Hip flexors, gluteus maximus, hamstrings, quads, hip adductors

Turn your back to the wall of the pool and brace yourself with your arms on the edge of the pool, deck, or gutter. Lift your hips and legs and begin shallow kicking with straight legs. In all kicking exercises (17 through 21), count one repetition each time your right foot breaks the surface of the water.

Exercise 18. Bicycling

Hamstrings, hip flexors, gluteus maximus, quads, hip adductors

Bend your knees and kick in a bicycling movement. For maximum benefit, lift the knee as close to the chest as possible, raise the foot well out of the water, and pull the heel in close to the buttock at the end of each kick (Photo 18).

18

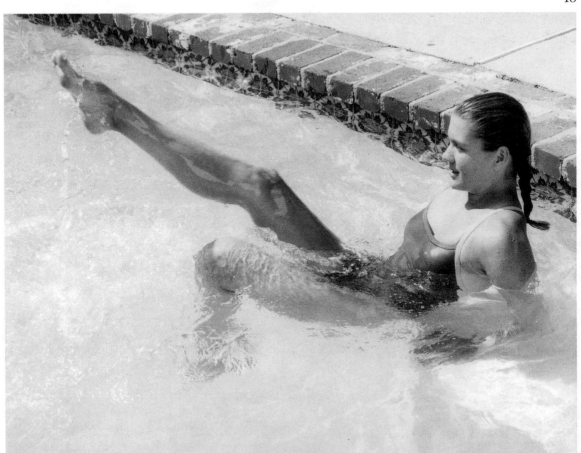

Exercise 19. Straight-Leg Deep Kick

Hip flexors, gluteus maximus, quads, hamstrings, hip adductors

If you have lower back pain, try this exercise slowly and with a narrow range of motion. If you don't experience any pain, proceed at a normal pace and increase the distance between the legs.

Straighten both knees as you lift your right leg to the water's surface and push the left leg toward the pool bottom (Photo 19). Moving with strength, change leg positions so the right leg sweeps toward the pool bottom and the left leg reaches toward the surface.

19

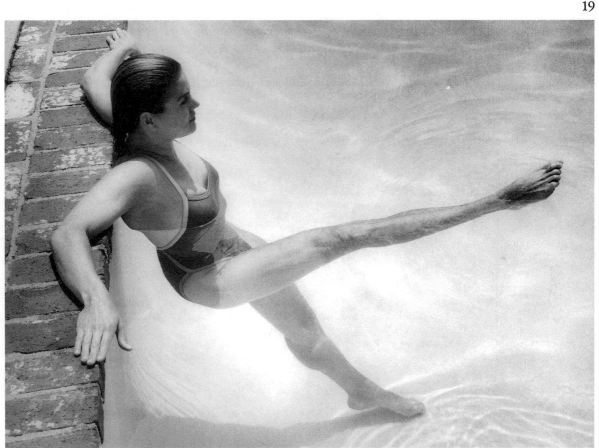

Exercise 20. Front Flutter Kick
Gluteus maximus, hip flexors, quads, hamstrings

Turn around and brace yourself facing the side of the pool. Hold the pool lip or gutter with one hand and place the other hand a foot lower to provide maximum leverage for maintaining this position. Lowering one hand also takes pressure off your lower back. Lift your hips and legs behind you and begin shallow straight-leg kicking. Photo 21 shows the correct hand placement.

Exercise 21. Slap Kick
Quads, hamstrings

With your body in the same position as in Exercise 20, bend your right knee so the heel lifts almost to the buttock (Photo 21). Then slap the top of your right foot against the surface of the water as your left heel lifts toward the buttock.

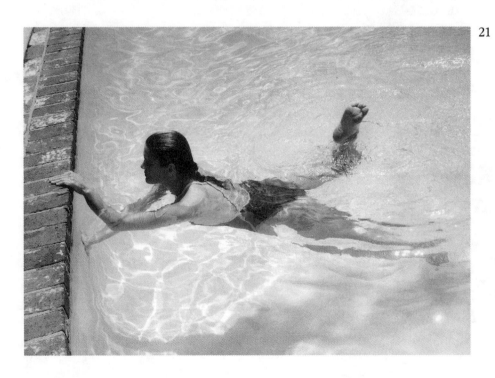

21

The
Complete
Waterpower
Workout
Book

110

If you remained in deep water for exercises 14 through 21, you should remove your flotation device for the remainder of the exercises. Your back can now push snugly against the pool wall. If you are a nonswimmer, perform these exercises in shallow water.

Exercise 22. Scissors

Hip abductors and adductors, abdominals, hip flexors, lats

Take the position in Photo 22A letting your lower back rest against the pool wall. Extend both legs straight out in front of you and open them sideways. With a scissors motion, cross one leg over the top of the other (Photo 22B). Open them, then continue crossing and opening them, alternating the top leg. Use as much force in opening the legs as you use in closing them.

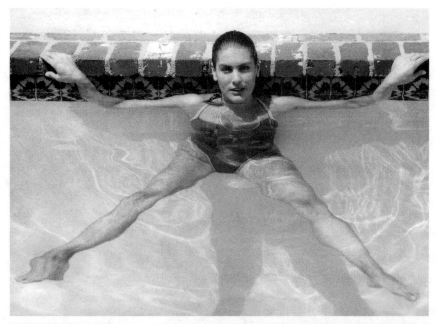

22A

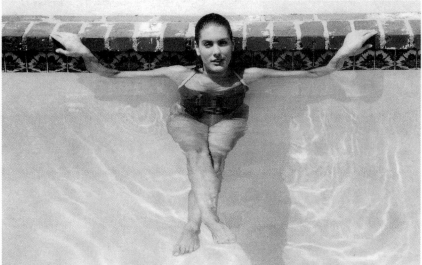

22B

Exercise 23. Pendulum

Abdominal obliques, hip flexors, lats, hip abductors and adductors, quads

Stay braced against the pool wall as in the previous exercise and hold both legs together straight in front of you. **If this hurts your lower back, bend the knees.** Keep your eyes focused straight ahead and don't move your head or upper body. Swing both legs as far as you can to the right (Photo 23), then back to the left. Your contact with the pool wall will rock from one hip to the other. Each sideways swing counts as one rep.

23

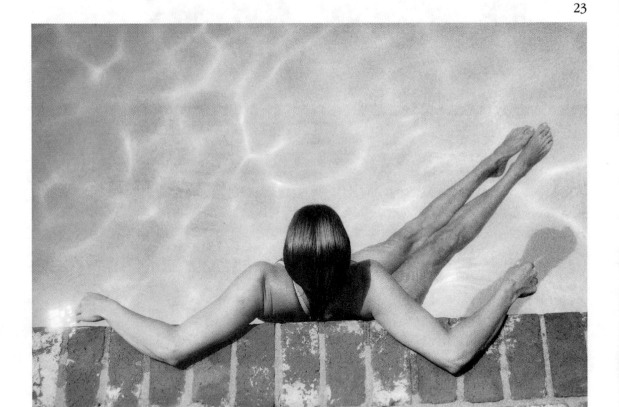

Exercise 24. Dips
Triceps, pecs, deltoids, lats, wrist flexors

If your pool has a gutter or railing, grasp it with fingers facing forward. If not, place your hands palms down on the deck in the most comfortable position you can establish. Now jump up and straighten your elbows, supporting yourself as in Photo 24A. From this position, lower yourself until the elbows reach a 90-degree bend (Photo 24B). Then push back up to the starting position.

If this exercise is too difficult for you, be content for several weeks with holding yourself steadily in the starting position. Over the coming weeks, you will be able to dip yourself to the low position. Begin with several reps, then gradually increase the number.

24A

24B

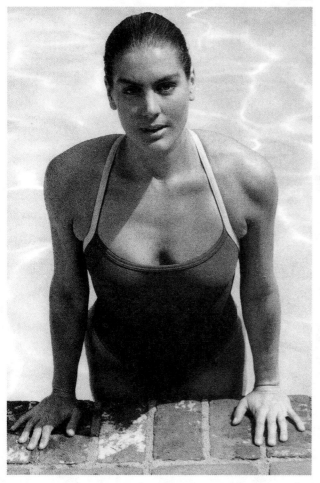
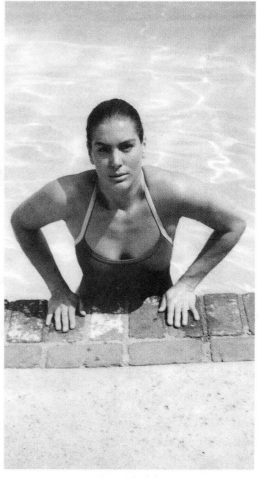

Exercise 25. Quad Stretch
Quads

Brace yourself by holding on to the side of the pool with your right hand. If you are in deep water, touch your right foot to the side of the pool for stability. Grasp your left ankle in your left hand and slowly pull the left heel toward the buttocks as in Photo 25. Keep the knees close together and maintain a "neutral" pelvis position (see Photos A and B, page 77). Never force a stretch if there is pain. Stretch only to the point of discomfort, ease back a bit, then hold the position until the muscles have relaxed and lengthened. Breathe deeply to increase the stretching process. Repeat on the right leg, holding on to the side of the pool with your left hand.

25

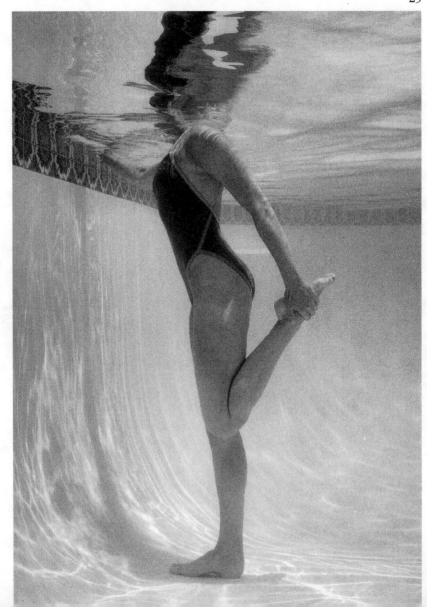

The
Complete
Waterpower
Workout
Book

114

Exercise 26. Hamstring Stretch

Hamstrings, gluteals, erector spinae, rhomboids, trapezius

Grasp a gutter, ladder, or side of the pool with both hands and place your right foot, toes up, against the pool wall as in Photo 26. If you are in deep water, your left leg dangles below. Keep your neck, shoulders, upper back, and arms relaxed as you try to straighten your right knee and try to push your right heel to make contact with the pool wall. Inhale and exhale deeply five times, then repeat on the left leg.

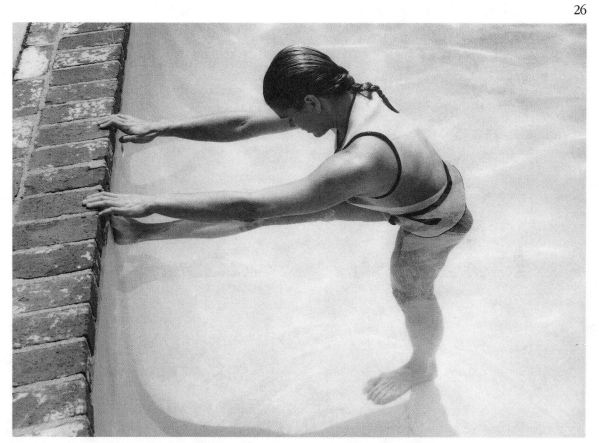

If you tend to become chilled toward the end of the workout, wear a Wet Wrap.

Exercise 27. Curl and Stretch

Erector spinae, trapezius, rhomboids, lats, hamstrings, gluteus maximus, gastroc/soleus complex

Continue holding the ladder or gutter. If your pool has neither, use Hol-Tite Restrainers (Photos 27A and 27B), grasp the pool's edge at the skimmer box or hold the lip of the pool deck. Bend both knees, placing your feet on a rung of the ladder or on the side of the pool. Curl up as tightly as you can, tucking your chin to your chest and pushing your tailbone down toward your heels (Photo 27A). Inhale and exhale slowly three to five times as you completely relax your neck, shoulders, back, and legs. Now slowly straighten your legs (Photo 27B). Hold this position for five long, slow breaths, keeping your shoulders and arms as relaxed as possible. Although the photos show a flotation belt, this is easily performed without one.

27A

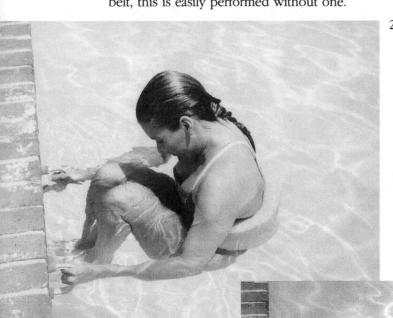

27B

The
Complete
Waterpower
Workout
Book

116

Exercise 28. Body Swing

Hip adductors and abductors, hamstrings, hip rotators, gastroc/soleus complex, lats, biceps, triceps, quads

Continue gripping the gutter, ladder, skimmer box, or Hol-Tite Restrainers. Open your feet to slightly more than shoulder width apart (Photo 28A). Now bend your right knee as far as you can and swing your body to the right, fully straightening the left knee (Photo 28B). Swing back to the left by straightening your right knee and fully bending your left. Swing back and forth five to ten times, taking time to enjoy this pleasurable stretch.

28A

28B

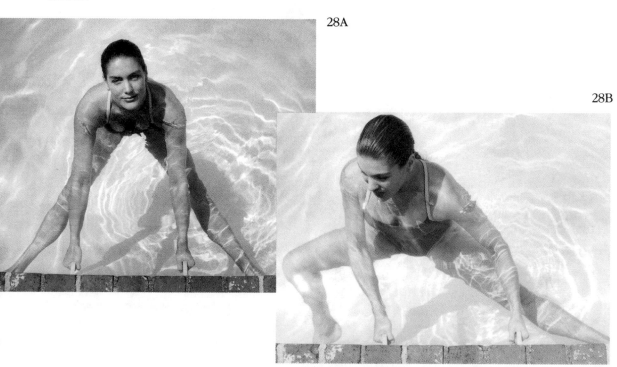

After your workout, relax and ask yourself these questions:

1. At what point or points did I begin to tire?
2. What exercises were particularly difficult? Should I hire a personal coach to learn the correct form?
3. Was there pain with any exercise?
4. Could I have put more effort—speed, power, precision—into the exercises?

The answers to these questions will help you plan your next Deep Waterpower Workout. Decide what level of effort you want to commit to your next workout and *do it*. If you experienced pain during the workout, read chapters 7 through 11 to learn how to modify this basic program to fit your specific needs.

The Deep Waterpower Workout

Level I: 20 reps   *Level II: 30 reps*   *Level III: 40 reps*

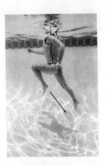

1. Water Running
Three-minute warm-up

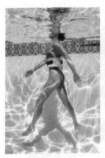

Basic walking   *Power walking*

2. Water Walking
Three-minute warm-up

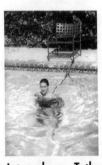

3. Intervals on Tether
Nine to twelve minutes
Water run, Speed walk, Power walk

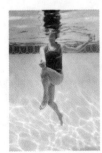 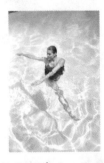 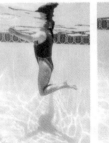

4. Bent-Knee Twist   **5. Straight-Leg Twist**   **6. Heel Lifts**

The
Complete
Waterpower
Workout
Book

118

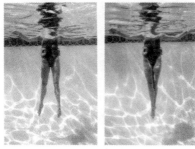

7. Quick Scissors

Alternate the front foot

8. Intervals

Nine to twelve minutes

Water run, Speed walk, Power walk

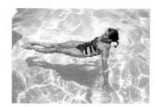 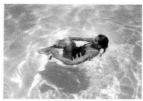 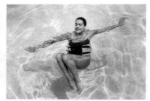

Straight **9. Abdominals** *Obliques variation*

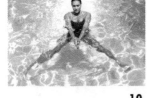 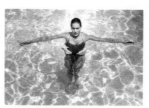

10. Flies **11. V-Kicks**

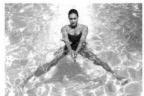

13. Intervals

Six to ten minutes

Water run, Speed walk, Power walk

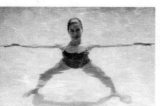 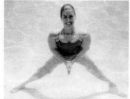

12. Back Kicks **14. Up/Down Pull**

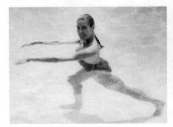 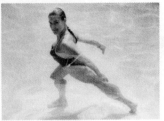

15. Dig Deep

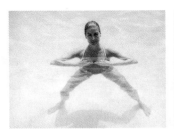 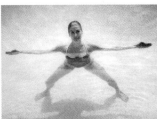

17. Back Flutter Kick

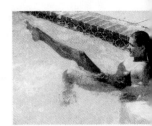

16. Arm Curls

18. Bicycling

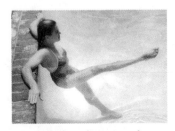 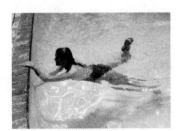

20. Front Flutter Kick

19. Straight-Leg Kick

21. Slap Kick

The
Complete
Waterpower
Workout
Book

120

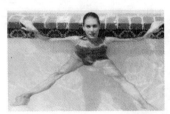 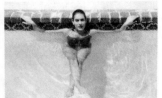

22. Scissors
Alternate top leg

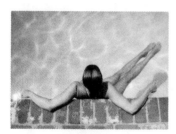

23. Pendulum

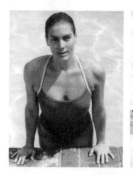

24. Dips

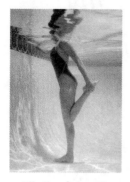

25. Quad Stretch
One rep each side

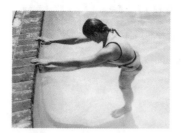

26. Hamstring Stretch
One rep each side

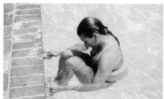
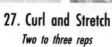

27. Curl and Stretch
Two to three reps

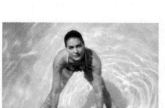
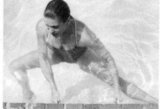

28. Body Swing
Six to eight reps each side

The Deep
Waterpower
Workout

Dance-Specific Waterpower Workouts

The
Complete
Waterpower
Workout
Book

122

D ancers are athletes as well as artists. During practice or performance, their finely tuned bodies are always in danger of an accident or a momentary loss of control or sudden weakness as they try to defy the laws of physics. So like all athletes, they must systematically develop the nine aspects of fitness: flexibility, aerobic capacity, anaerobic capacity, musculoskeletal resiliency, strength, power, speed, skill—and they must *rest,* for like other athletes, they must push their limits without overtraining. Dancers, like athletes, are beginning to follow a hard/easy scheme of training as well as principles of periodization. (See Chapter 1.)

Dance-Specific Waterpower Workouts allow dancers to *add* training hours to their regimen because their extra leaps, bounds, and jumps use water as a landing cushion. Water spares dancers' bodies any additional trauma.

Waterpower can also be used *instead of* dance sessions. Whenever a small strain or pain makes a dancer leery of working at full power or speed in the studio, the practice session can move to the pool.

When you enter the water, you will notice a tendency to relax. Yet you must strive to pierce the water as you pierce the air in a dance studio even though piercing water requires more energy. Notice, too, that if your form is not exact, incorrect movement will throw you off your center of balance. Because of this, training in water actually helps you improve your technique.

Before every session, sit on the side of the pool or on a step and perform ten ankle circles in each direction. For the warm-up you have both a shallow and a deep-water option. Healthy dancers can choose either. Injured dancers should start in deep water to avoid all impact. Turn to pages 85 and 86 for help in selecting a flotation device. Once outfitted, slip into the pool and begin the deep warm-up. After the shallow or deep warm-up, all dancers go to the side of the pool for an extended stretch and barre work. Next come specific dance moves to help you retain your timing. Then finish your workout with the remainder of The Waterpower Workout or Deep Waterpower Workout. Some exercises are the standard version; others are modified for dancers. The primary muscle movers are listed. Although the abdominal and abdominal oblique muscles are not listed, they work powerfully in virtually all exercises to stabilize the torso so that the muscles of the extremities have a solid base to pull against.

A

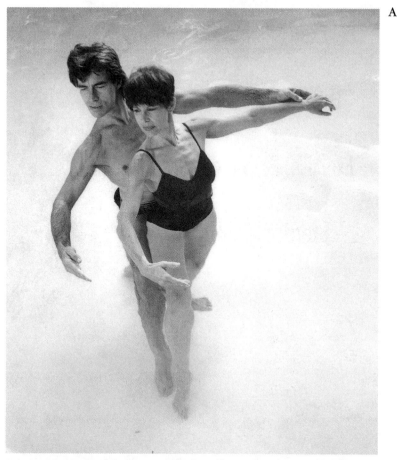

Dancers/choreographers Jacqui and Bill Landrum often train in the water together.

Ballet dancers normally execute their moves in a turnout position of the feet and legs that can often lead to complications of the knee and hip joints. But dancers who have used Waterpower report that by doing the exercises in both turnout and parallel positions, they create a more balanced strength in the thigh, buttocks, and hip area and therefore experience less pain in the hip and the knee. So when doing your Dance-Specific Waterpower Workout, begin each exercise as it appears in the basic program. The toes point straight forward and the feet are parallel to one another. Then when you have completed half your repetitions, switch to a turnout position to finish the other half.

Warm-Up——Shallow

In exercises 1 through 3, perform half of your repetitions with the feet parallel, then complete your reps with the feet and legs turned out.

Exercise 1. Lunges *(Exercise 1, page 36)*

Exercise 2. Crossovers *(Exercise 2, page 37)*

Exercise 3. Squat Jumps *(Exercise 3, page 38)*

Exercise 4. V Kicks *(Exercise 8, page 43)*

The
Complete
Waterpower
Workout
Book

124

Warm-Up—Deep

Exercise 1. Water Running *(Exercise 1, page 88)*

Warm up for three to five minutes working on what might be a new movement. Many dancers don't run, so take time to learn and perfect good form.

Exercise 2. Water Walking *(Exercise 2, page 90)*

This exercise will feel more dancelike to you, although you should begin with the feet parallel. To add extra work to the calf muscles, try the power-walk technique, flexing the foot as the leg swings forward, then pointing the foot as the leg swings back. Water walk two minutes with the feet parallel, then switch to turnout and continue two minutes more.

Exercise 3. Intervals—Set 1 *(Exercise 3, page 92)*

Water running—the same.
Water walking—alternate between a parallel and turnout foot position.

Exercise 4. Développé Splits

Hip adductors and abductors, hip flexors, gluteus maximus, hip rotators,
hamstrings, quads, deltoids, pecs, teres, rhomboids, lats

Assume the position in Photo 4A, feet together below your body. Now place your hands in preparatory position in front. Then stretch the right foot forward and the left foot back to reach the position shown in Photo 4B. Although the photos don't show the arm action, your left arm is forward, right arm back. Return both feet and both arms to the starting position. Now reach the left foot forward and right arm forward, the right foot and left arm backward. Each right/left cycle equals one repetition.

4A

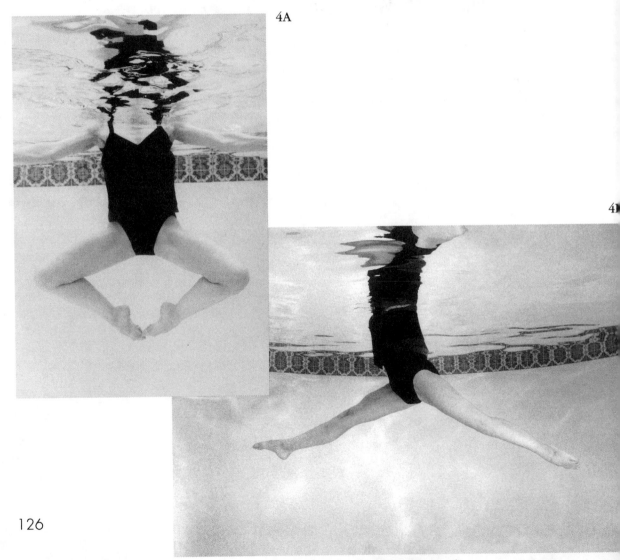

4I

126

(Wet Belt pictured)

Dance Work

Now that you have warmed up, move to the shallow end of the pool. If an injury requires extra buoyancy protection, continue wearing your flotation device. If an injury is relatively minor and you can perform all dance movements in water with no pain, remove the flotation device.

The nonimpact exercises are presented first; those that follow add increasingly higher degrees of impact. If you feel any pain at the site of your injury, backtrack to the previous exercise and wait until the next session before trying, even more gently, again.

Move to the side of the pool to perform exercises 5 through 14, dance stretches and technique work. If you have a railing in your pool, terrific. If not, use the side of the pool or a ledge.

Forcing turnout to an extreme may be dangerous, because the ability to turn out varies and is based on the structure of your body. Determine your own safe turnout position in this way: Stand with your ankles touching, feet parallel. Let your weight fall back onto your heels, tighten your buttocks, then turn both feet out simultaneously. This is your natural and safe turnout position. Don't try to force beyond this position while performing the following exercises. Note: Within a workout, be consistent and do each exercise first on one side, then the other, as you would in class. Instructions are written as if you were beginning with your left hand holding on to the poolside, but the photos show exercises executed on both the left and the right sides.

Exercise 5. Fourth-Position Extended Barre Stretch

Hamstrings, hip rotators, hip adductors, erector spinae, deltoids, trapezius, quads, gastroc/soleus complex, lats, abdominals, gluteus maximus, hip flexors, pecs

Assume your safe turnout position. Place your left leg on the bar or side of the pool, keeping your hips and shoulders squared toward the left leg. The ankle of your left leg is in line with your nose. Gently *plié* your left leg into a front attitude and slowly lean your upper body forward, reaching your nose toward your toes. Take two deep breaths as you stretch. Now stand erect and extend your left leg, trying to touch your little toe to the side of the pool or bar. Keep your left leg in this position as you move your right leg through these positions: *demi-plié,* straighten, *relevé,* lower the heel. Do this four times. Next, raise your left arm into an overhead fifth position and *port de bras* forward (Photo 5A), *combré* back (Photo 5B), *port de bras* forward, *combré* back. Do this also four times. Finally, rotate your trunk and your left arm to your left as the right shoulder moves forward. Your hips don't move. Hold for two long, slow breaths. Repeat this entire sequence standing on your left leg, your right leg on the bar or side of the pool.

5A

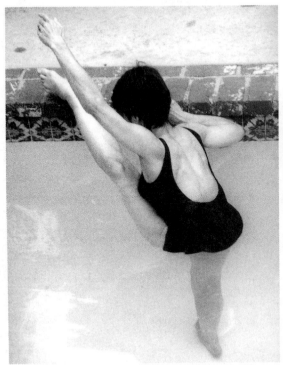

5B

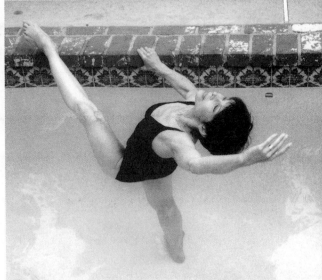

To move to second position for Exercise 6, *relevé* on your left foot and promenade your left heel into second position, keeping your weight directly over your left leg.

Exercise 6. Second-Position Extended Barre Stretch

Hamstrings, hip adductors and abductors, hip rotators, gluteus maximus, quads, deltoids, lats, abdominals, abdominal obliques, pecs, quadratus lumborum, gastroc/soleus complex

Stand in second position with your right leg on the bar or side of the pool. *Demi-plié*, keeping your weight directly over your left leg. Keep your hips square and push them toward the side of the pool (Photo 6A). *Port de bras* your left arm up and over to position 6B. Press your left hip down as though both buttocks are sitting on the edge of a bench. Feel your shoulder pulling away from your hip. Reach up and back to the starting position. *Port à bras* your right arm up and over, then back to the starting position. Move from *demi-plié* to a straight left leg and repeat the *port de bras* with each arm. Then repeat once more from *relevé*.

Next, place your right hand on the side of the pool in front of your left shoulder and twist your upper body so that your left arm reaches over your head toward your right foot. Breathe deeply several times. Repeat the entire sequence standing on your right leg, your left leg on the bar or side of the pool.

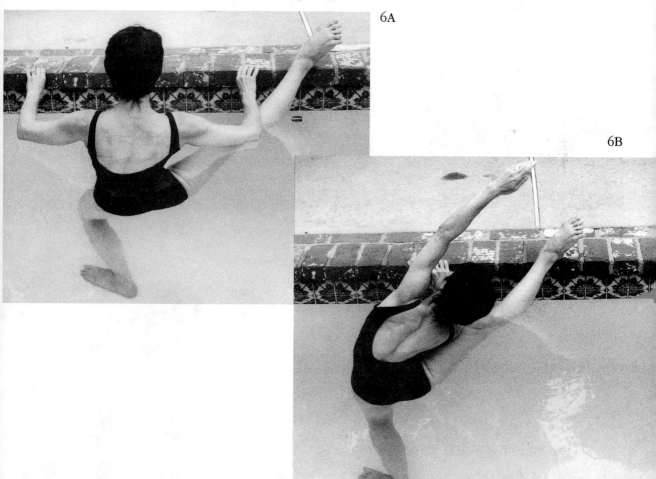

6A

6B

Exercise 7. Demi-Plié and Grand Plié

Quads, hip adductors, hip rotators, hamstrings, gluteus maximus, gastroc/soleus complex

If you have a knee injury, save this exercise for last.

Stand with your left hand resting on the bar or side of the pool. Center your weight equally over both feet in first position. Hold your torso and head erect, knees turned outward in a direct line over the feet. Bend both knees and descend to *demi-plié* as shown in Photo 7A; press through both heels against the floor and rise to the starting position. Repeat eight times. Now perform eight *grands pliés,* descending to position 7B.

7A

7B

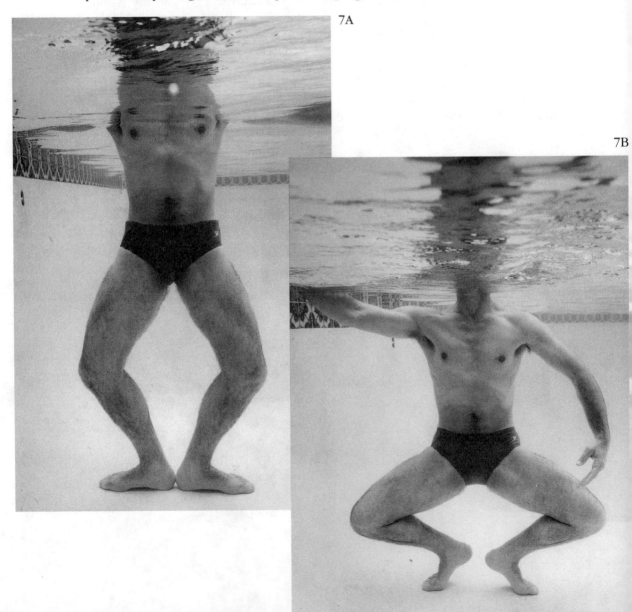

Exercise 8. Tendu

Hip flexors, hip rotators, quads, gluteus maximus, hamstrings, hip adductors, gastroc/soleus complex

Continue standing in first position, holding the bar or pool with your left hand. This exercise is composed of four rapid, strong movements that require powerful muscle contractions. Sharply thrust your right foot forward to position 8A, keeping your toe in contact with the pool bottom. Then with another quick movement, lift and hold the leg at 45 degrees (Photo 8B). Quickly press the leg back to *tendu*. Finally, emphasize the pull back to the starting position. Move four times with quickness and control through the following: (1) *tendu,* (2) reach, (3) *tendu,* (4) close. Perform four more series like this to the side and then to the back. Turn so that your right hand now holds the bar or pool and repeat the entire sequence with your left leg.

8A 8B

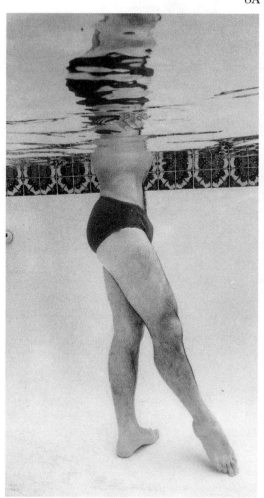
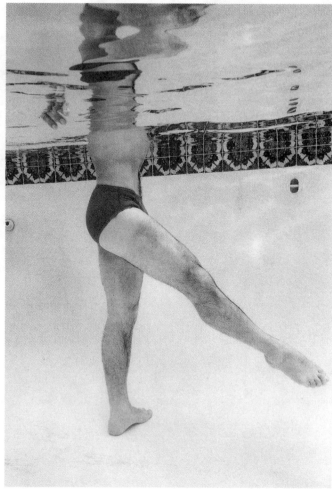

Exercise 9. Dégagé

Hip flexors, hip rotators, quads, gluteus maximus, hamstrings, hip adductors, tibialis anterior, gastroc/soleus complex

Turn back so your left hand holds the bar or pool as you continue to stand in first position. Your weight should be evenly distributed over both feet. Point your toes and sharply lift your right leg straight forward to 45 degrees. (Photo 9A.) Flex the foot (Photo 9B) and pull the heel down to the pool bottom to first position. Do four repetitions of: (1) point and lift, (2) flex and pull down. Repeat *en croix* (front, side, and back). Then turn 180 degrees and perform the same sequence with your left leg.

9A

9B

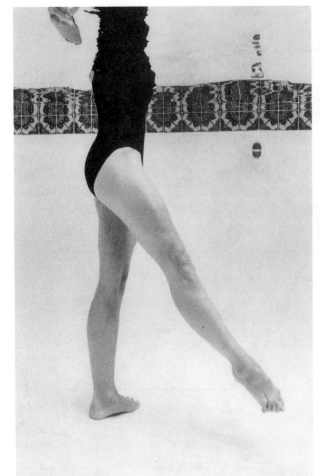

Exercise 10. Passé

Hip flexors, sartorius, quads, hamstrings, hip rotators, hip abductors and adductors, tensor fasciae latae, gastroc/soleus complex

Turn so your left hand holds the bar or pool. From first position, bend your right knee and raise your pointed right foot to the left knee (Photo 10A). Extend the right foot straight forward to the position shown in Photo 10B. Now pull the right foot back to the knee, then swing it laterally to the position shown in Photo 10C. Do eight reps on each leg.

10A

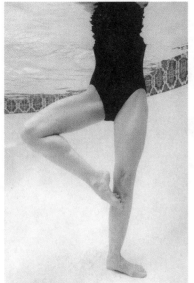

10B

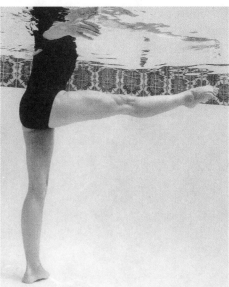

10C

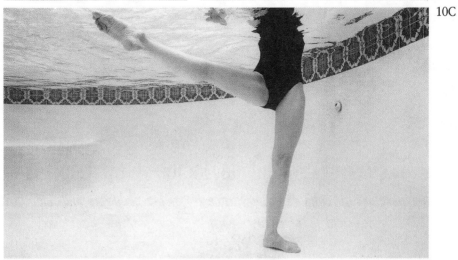

In *rond de jambe* exercises 11 through 13, remember to lead with your heel and drop your tailbone down so your hips remain totally square throughout the movement.

Exercise 11. Rond de Jambe à Terre

Hip flexors, sartorius, hip rotators, tensor fasciae latae, hip abductors and adductors, quads, gluteus maximus, hamstrings, gastroc/soleus complex, tibialis anterior

En dehors (outward): Stand in first position with your right hand holding the bar or side of the pool. Keep your right leg straight as the left foot extends forward to a point directly in front of your nose. Describe a half circle on the bottom of the pool (Photo 11A) with the foot ending at the back (Photo 11B). Then the left foot moves forward in a straight line. Your inner thighs brush together as the heel lowers to the bottom to pass through first position before beginning the next half circle. Complete four *ronds de jambes. En dehors* (outward): Reverse the direction of the half circle and perform four times.

11A

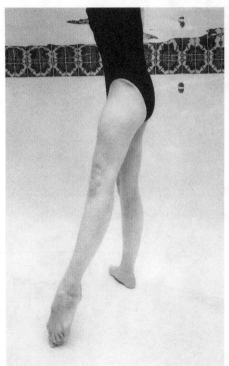

11B

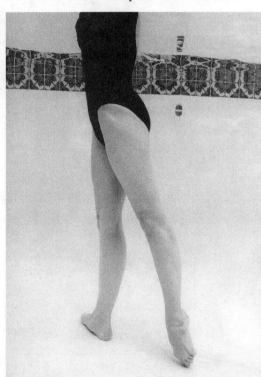

Exercise 12. Rond de Jambe—60 Degrees

Hip flexors, hip rotators, tensor fasciae latae, hip abductors and adductors, quads, gluteus maximus, hamstrings, gastroc/soleus complex

Repeat the sequence as in Exercise 11, but this time lift the foot away from the bottom of the pool to 60 degrees as you perform your half circles. Do four reps *en dehors* and four reps *en dedans.*

The
Complete
Waterpower
Workout
Book

134

Exercise 13. Grand Rond de Jambe en L'Air
Hip flexors, hip rotators, tensor fasciae latae, quads, hip abductors and adductors, gluteus maximus, hamstrings

Repeat the sequence as in Exercise 11, but this time lift the foot away from the bottom of the pool to 90 degrees (Photo 13A) as you perform your half circles. Keep your chest lifted as you tilt your pelvis forward to allow the hip to complete the rotation. (Photos 13B and 13C.) Do four reps *en dehors* and four reps *en dedans*.

13A

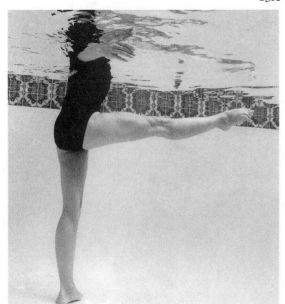

13B

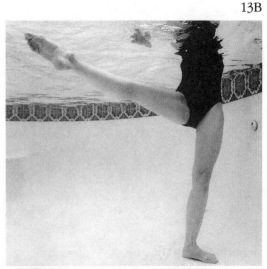

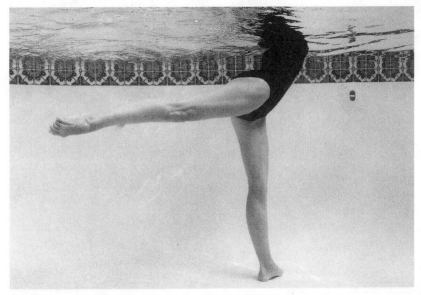

13C

Exercise 14. Fondu Développé Relevé

Quads, hip flexors, sartorius, tensor fasciae latae, hip adductors and abductors, gluteus maximus, hamstrings, gastroc/soleus complex, erector spinae, deltoids, trapezius, rhomboids, lats

Skip this exercise if you have a back injury.

Stand on your left leg with your right toe pointing in *coupé* in front of the left ankle (Photo 14A). *Demi-plié* on the left leg. Hold the hip stationary. Begin to rise from *demi-plié* as your right leg moves through attitude. Push all the way up to *relevé* on your left leg as your right leg lifts out of the water (Photo 14B). Retrace your movements back to *demi-plié* and *coupé*. Perform four to the front, four to the side, and four to the back (arabesque). As you perform the four to the back, tilt your torso forward to allow the height without hurting your back. Turn and perform four standing on your right leg *en croix*.

14A

14B

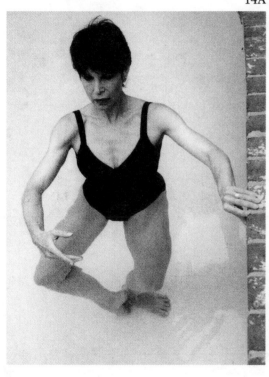
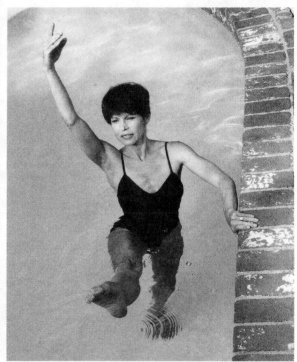

Exercise 15. Battements

Hip abductors and adductors, hip flexors, tensor fasciae latae, hamstrings, gluteals

Standing in first position (turnout), lift your right leg straight out to the side without altering the upper-body position (Photo 15A). Keep your hips square and concentrate on reaching down and out with the back of the leg. Pull the right leg back to the starting position. Do this four times. Repeat with the left leg.

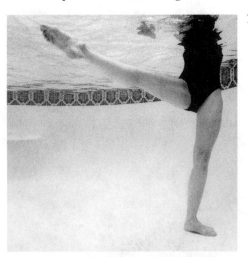

15A

Now turn the feet to a parallel position (Photo 15B), which allows you to focus on the abductors and adductors as well as balance the muscles surrounding the hip joint. Lift the left leg straight out to the side (Photo 15C), then pull back to the starting position. Perform four reps, then turn 180 degrees to work the right leg, also in this parallel position.

15B

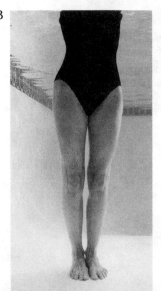

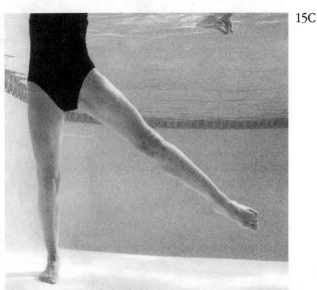

15C

After you have gained mastery of exercises 8 through 15 in water, you might try increasing resistance (work load) to induce further strength gains. Strap an Aquatoner onto your ankle (Photo 15D) (see page 230) or pull on a Hydro-Tone boot (see page 231).

15D

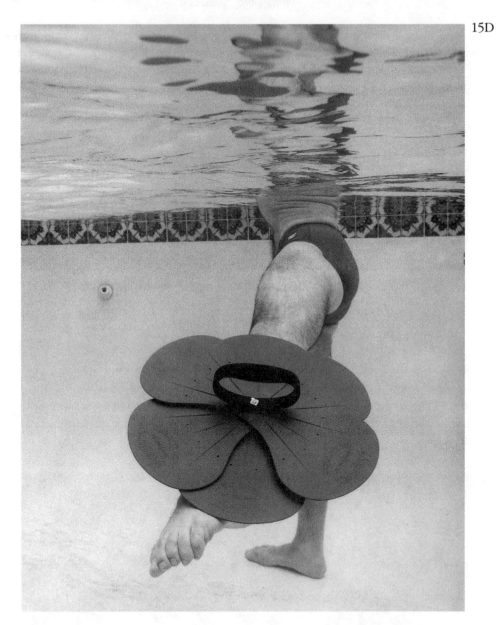

The
Complete
Waterpower
Workout
Book

138

Exercise 16. Echappés

*Gastroc/soleus complex, quads, gluteus maximus, hip rotators,
hip adductors and abductors, hamstrings*

**If yours is a calf, foot, or ankle injury, move this exercise to the end of the
series. Try it gently at first. If you experience sharp pain, wait until the next
session and try again, more gently. Try two reps, then three and four on
subsequent workouts.**

Stand in fifth position, right foot forward, knees turned out in a direct line over the
feet. Execute a *demi-plié* (Photo 16A), then spring onto the balls of your feet (Photo
16B). If you wear an old pair of toe shoes into the pool, you can spring onto your toes.
As you return to *demi-plié,* place the left foot in front. Perform ten to fifty reps, depending on your capability.

16A

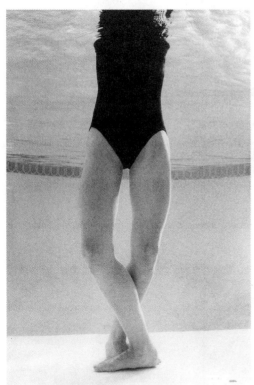 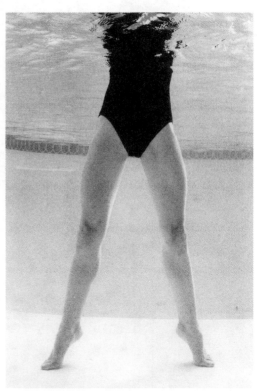

16B

Perform the dance movements that follow in chest-deep water, moving smoothly and
gently across the width of the pool. Lead with the right leg crossing the pool, then lead
with the left leg returning. Whenever more strenuous jumps are required, perform the
first crossing of the pool with the noninjured leg, concentrating on precise rhythm and
coordination. Then attempt to duplicate that coordination on the healing leg.

Exercise 17. Glissade

Quads, hip abductors and adductors, tensor fasciae latae, hamstrings, gluteus maximus, gastroc/soleus complex, deltoids, pecs, trapezius

Stand in fifth position with your right foot front and right shoulder forward (Photo 17). Arms are in preparatory position. Execute a *demi-plié*; slide your right foot along the floor to second position with the toe pointed. Open your arms a short distance to the sides. Push away from the floor with your left foot and transfer your weight onto your right foot. *Demi-plié* again, sliding back to fifth position returning your arms to preparatory position. Cross the pool several times with *glissades.* Face the same way so that you lead with opposite legs on each crossing.

17

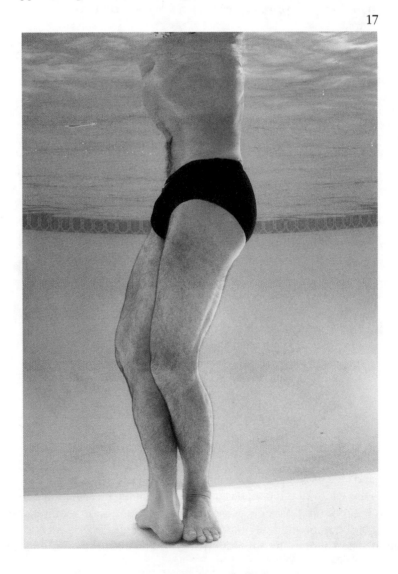

The
Complete
Waterpower
Workout
Book

140

Exercise 18. Chassé

Quads, gastroc/soleus complex, gluteus maximus, hamstrings, hip abductors and adductors

Stay in fifth position, right foot front and right shoulder forward. Hold arms either in second position with the hands on the surface of the water, or in an overhead fifth position. Execute a *demi-plié*; extend your pointed right foot to your right (Photo 18A). Slide right and transfer your weight to your right foot. Jump up, hit both legs together in *soussus* (Photo 18B), then land back in fifth position, preparing for another *demi-plié* and another *chassé*. Cross the pool leading with the right leg. Recross the pool leading with the left.

18A

18B

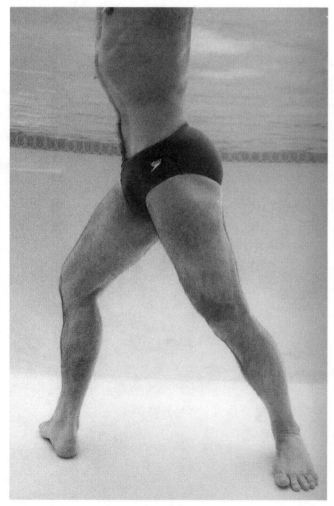
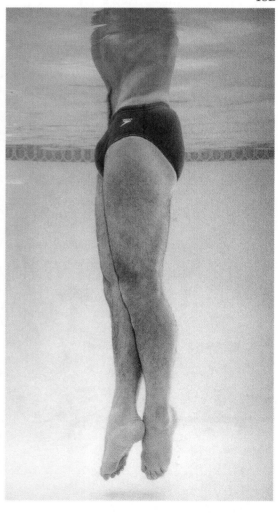

Exercise 19. Cecchetti Pas de Chat

Hip flexors, quads, tensor fasciae latae, hamstrings, gastroc/soleus complex, hip abductors and adductors, gluteus maximus

Start in fifth position with the left foot and shoulder forward. Arms are held in second position, hands on the surface of the water, or in an overhead fifth position throughout the exercise. *Demi-plié* on both feet, then lift the right foot sharply upward under the torso with the right knee turned out (Photo 19A). Immediately jump, lifting the left foot to replace the right one under the body. For a moment, both legs are bent beneath the body as it is suspended in the water (Photo 19B). The right foot returns to the pool bottom and is quickly followed by the left foot for a return to fifth position and a *demi-plié.* Your mental commands during this exercise are "Knee, knee." Think of lifting each knee to your armpit. Cross the pool leading with the right leg; recross leading with the left.

19A

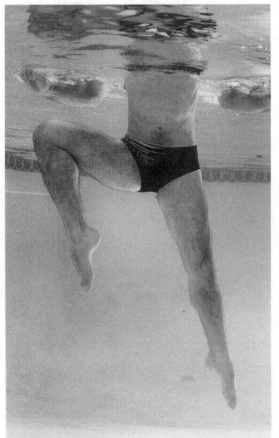

19B

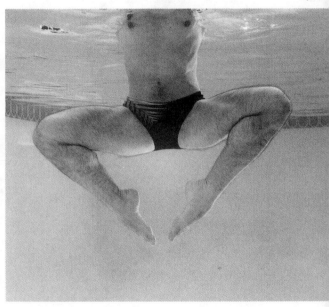

Exercise 20. Changement

*Quads, gastroc/soleus complex, hip abductors and adductors,
gluteus maximus, hamstrings*

Stand in fifth position, right foot front, arms in preparatory position. Execute a *demi-plié*, distributing your weight equally between the feet. Jump upward, straightening both legs to fifth position in the air. Change your left foot to the forward position. Toes strike the pool bottom first before lowering the heels into fifth position *demi-plié*, left foot forward. Repeat eight times, changing feet each time.

Exercise 21. Second and Fifth Tours

Hip rotators, hip abductors and adductors, quads, hamstrings,
gastroc/soleus complex, deltoids, rhomboids, abdominal obliques, teres, lats

Stand away from the side of the pool in fifth position, right foot forward. Your right arm is in pirouette position; your left arm is in second position at the surface of the water (Photo 21A). *Demi-plié,* then jump up, swinging your right arm to the right to help you execute a 180-degree turn. Land facing the opposite direction with your feet in second position, your arms out to the sides as in Photo 21B. Execute another 180-degree turn to your right as you pull your legs back to fifth position and your right arm back to the starting position. Complete four full circles before reversing and performing four more to your left.

21A

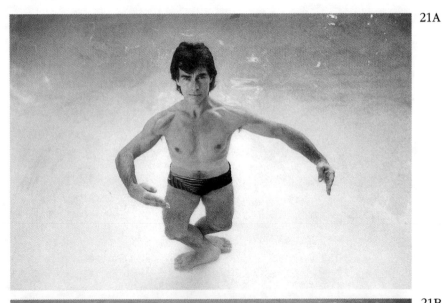

21B

The
Complete
Waterpower
Workout
Book

144

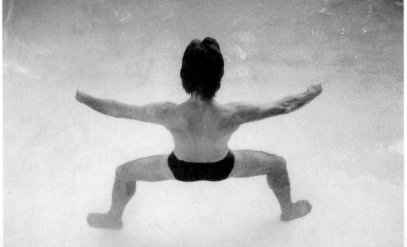

Exercise 22. Your Favorite Dance Combination

Put together a series of dance moves that please you and allow you to strengthen the weakened areas of your body. Repeat five times in one direction, then five times in the other.

Once again, you can choose between shallow and deep water for the rest of your workout. If you are injured, stick with the no-impact workout of deep water, then move to shallow water as soon as you can safely tolerate weight bearing.

Deep Waterpower Exercises

Now complete your pool workout with these Deep Waterpower exercises. Some of them remain the same as in Chapter 3. Others are modified as shown below.

Exercise 23. Bent-Knee Twist *(Exercise 4, page 94)*

Exercise 24. Straight-Leg Twist *(Exercise 5, page 95)*

Exercise 25. Heel Lifts *(Exercise 6, page 96)*

Exercise 26. Quick Scissors *(Exercise 7, page 97)*

Perform one quarter of your reps with toes pointed, feet parallel; one quarter with toes pointed and turned out; one quarter with feet flexed, parallel; and one quarter with feet flexed and turned out.

Exercise 27. Intervals—Set 2 *(Exercise 8, page 98)*

Water running—the same.

Water walking—alternate between a parallel and a turnout foot position.

Exercise 28. Abdominals *(Exercise 9, page 100)*

Exercise 29. Flies *(Exercise 10, page 101)*

Perform half your reps with feet parallel and half with feet turned out.

Exercise 30. V Kicks *(Exercise 11, page 102)*

Exercise 31. Back Kicks *(Exercise 12, page 103)*

Perform half your reps with feet parallel and half with feet turned out. Stretch any muscles that feel tight, then do a second set, this time doing a left/right repetition in the parallel position, then a left/right rep in turnout. Alternate between the two foot positions, noting the different gluteal muscles at work in each exercise.

Waterpower Exercises

Once you can perform all the shallow-water impact exercises (16 through 22), you may wish to finish your workout in shallow water as well. In that case, do the following exercises from The Waterpower Workout (Chapter 2) to replace exercises 23 through 31 above. Do the first half of your reps with feet in a parallel position. Complete the last half of your reps with feet in a turnout position.

Exercise 23. Side-Straddle Jumps *(Exercise 5, page 40)*

The
Complete
Waterpower
Workout
Book

146

Exercise 24. Front-Straddle Jumps *(Exercise 7, page 42)*

Exercise 25. Double Heel Lifts *(Exercise 9, page 44)*

Exercise 26. Rocking Horse *(Exercise 10, page 45)*

Exercise 27. Leg Swings *(Exercise 11, page 46)*

Exercise 28. Front Kicks *(Exercise 12, page 47)*

Exercise 29. Back Kicks *(Exercise 13, page 48)*

Perform half your reps with feet parallel and half with feet turned out. Stretch any muscles that feel tight, then do a second set, this time doing a left/right repetition in the parallel position then a left/right rep in turnout. Alternate between the two foot positions, noting the different gluteal muscles at work in each exercise.

Exercise 30. Power Frog Jumps *(Exercise 14, page 49)*

Perform half your reps with knees forward, then the last half your reps with knees wide to the side.

Exercise 31. One-Legged Frog Jumps *(Exercise 15, page 50)*

Perform one third your reps with the bent knee forward; one third with the bent knee to the side; then the final one third with a straight leg out to the side.

Dance-Specific Waterpower Workouts

Deep

Shallow

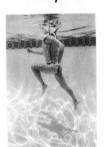

OR

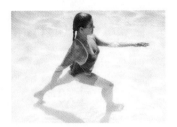

1. Water Running

1. Lunges
parallel
turned out

Basic Walk   *Power Walk*

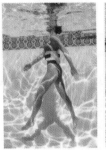

OR

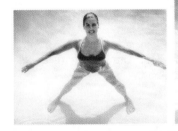

2. Water Walking
parallel
turned out

2. Cross-Overs
parallel
turned out

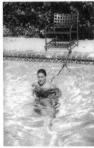

OR

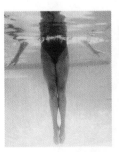

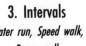

The
Complete
Waterpower
Workout
Book

148

3. Intervals
Water run, Speed walk,
Power walk

3. Squat Jumps
parallel
turned out

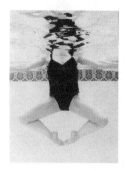
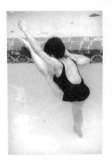

OR

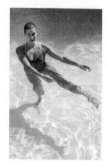

4. Développé Splits

4. V-Kicks

Dance work

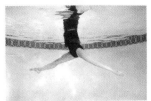
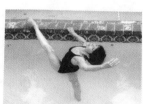

5. Fourth-Position Extended Barre Stretch

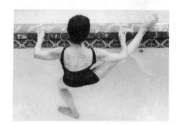
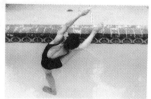

6. Second-Position Extended Barre Stretch

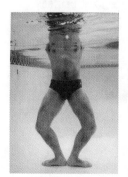
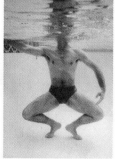

7. Demi-Pliés and Grand Pliés

Dance-Specific
Waterpower
Workouts

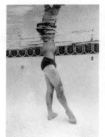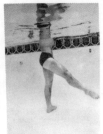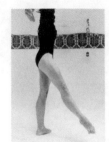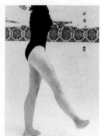

8. Tendu

9. Dégagé

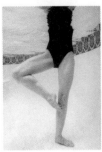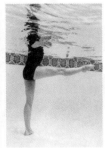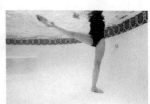

10. Passé

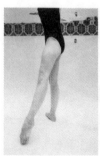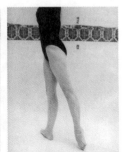

11. Rond de Jambe À Terre

12. Rond de Jambe—Sixty Degrees

The
Complete
Waterpower
Workout
Book

150

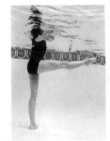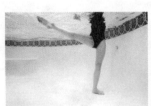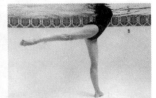

13. Grand Rond de Jambe en L'air

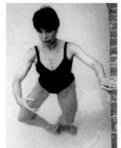
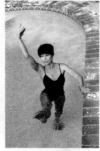

14. Fondu Développé Releve

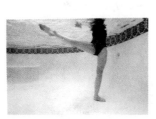
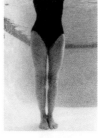
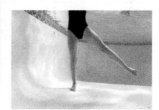

15. Battement

turned out
parallel

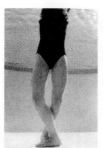
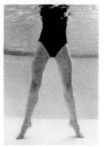
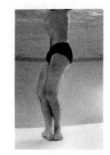

16. Echappé   17. Glissade

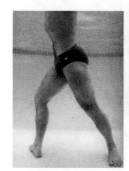
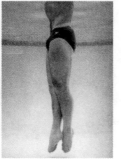
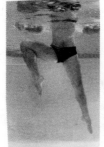
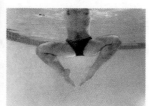

18. Chassé   19. Cecchetti Pas de Chat

20. Changement

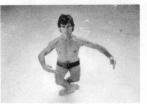

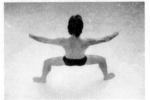

22. Your Favorite Dance Combination

21. Second and Fifth Tours

| **Deep Waterpower Exercises** | **Waterpower Exercises** |

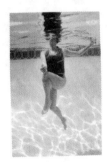

OR

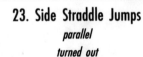

23. Bent-Knee Twist

23. Side Straddle Jumps
parallel
turned out

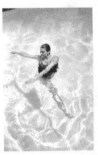

OR

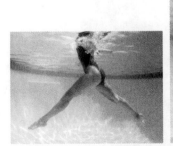

24. Straight-Leg Twist

24. Front Straddle Jumps
parallel
turned out

The
Complete
Waterpower
Workout
Book

152

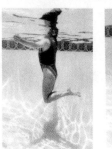 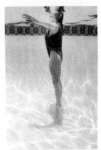

OR

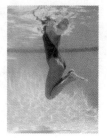

25. Heel Lifts

25. Heel Lifts

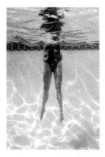 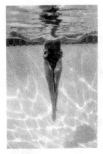

OR

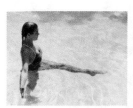 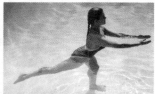

26. Quick Scissors
point + parallel
flex + parallel
point + turnout
flex + turnout

26. Rocking Horse
parallel
turned out

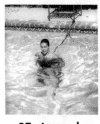

OR

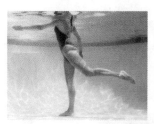 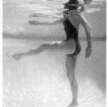

27. Intervals
Water run, speed walk,
power walk

27. Leg Swings
parallel
turned out

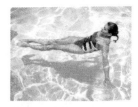 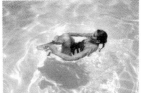 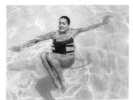

OR

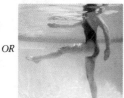

standard   *variation*

28. Abdominals

28. Front Kicks
parallel
turned out

153

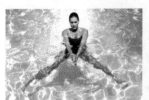 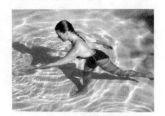

OR

29. Flies
Feet parallel
turned out

29. Back Kicks
parallel
turned out

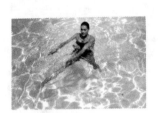 *OR*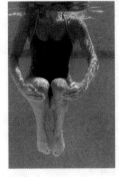

30. V-Kicks

30. Power Frog Jumps
knees forward
knees out to sides

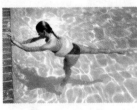 *OR*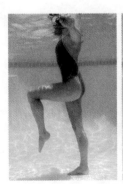

31. Back Kicks
parallel
turned out

31. One-Legged Frog Jumps
knee forward
knee to side
straight leg to side

The
Complete
Waterpower
Workout
Book

154

F i v e

Sport-Specific Waterpower Workouts

I f you want to run fast, you have to run fast. If you want to kick hard, you have to kick hard. If you want to swim long, you have to swim long. No matter what the sport, sooner or later you must approach full speed, full strength, full distance in your training. High-speed, high-impact, or long-distance repetitions often cause injuries, so athletes and coaches walk a fine line when scheduling workout and rest periods. They must find a way to complete the necessary training without crossing the line into overtraining. They must reach and sustain high velocity without overstressing the speed mechanisms. They must learn to recruit the maximum number of muscle fibers for top strength without straining fragile connective tissue. They must teach the body's endurance systems to continue working even when muscle fuel feels as though it has been depleted.

On land, such high-level training is limited. Only a few precision sprints can be performed before fatigue endangers the sprinter. Only a dozen or so kicks can send the football through the goalposts before the kicker's leg must be protected. Only so many miles can be logged by the marathoner before there's a chance of stress damage. But in the water, athletes can run, jump, and kick over and over again without fear of injury.

Sport-Specific Waterpower Workouts began at the International Sportsmedicine Institute (ISI) in 1983 in response to the rehabilitation needs of injured elite athletes gathering in Los Angeles for pre-Olympic competitions. French pole-vaulters; Greek javelin throwers; Cuban sprinters, hurdlers, and discus throwers; Kenyan distance runners; and dozens of other athletes came to ISI for treatment of their injuries and also found a new rehabilitative tool that helped them maintain their world-class fitness level while their injuries healed.

At first most coaches and athletes merely considered these water workouts an effective emergency cross-training tool—something to keep the athlete active and sane during rehabilitation. But soon some outstanding stories of success began to emerge: Mary Decker Slaney set a world record at 2,000 meters after a month in the pool and only one land workout prior to the race. Joan Benoit Samuelson won a gold medal in the marathon after doing Waterpower workouts to protect her postsurgical knee. Jeanette Bolden trained strictly in water because of a broken foot, raced in the 1984 Olympic Games on that broken foot, won a gold medal in the 400-meter relay, then had a cast placed on her foot after the race. Athletes were being restored to their winning ways with Waterpower. They were actually getting *stronger* during their rehabilitation periods. This new water-training component was needed in their basic fitness plan. With it, they discovered yet another tool to help them hold together their year-round training programs.

In this way, water training has become standard practice in the training of elite athletes. No longer are athletes or coaches waiting for injury to strike to turn to the water. Now they are incorporating Waterpower into their existing training schedules. The more progressive coaches, such as Bobby Kersee and Randy Huntington, understand the value of cross training athletes *before* an injury happens. Whenever they sense an injury coming, they immediately switch their star runners and jumpers—Mike Powell, Florence Griffith Joyner, Gail Devers, Gea Johnson, Valerie Brisco, Jackie Joyner-Kersee—from the track to the pool, while asking that they do the same workout in the water that they had scheduled that day for land.

Waterpower lets athletes take a day off without taking a day off.

Increase Speed, Improve Technique, Learn Key Positions

The
Complete
Waterpower
Workout
Book

156

You can focus on speed and anaerobic capacity by adding Waterpower sprints to your routine. You will be able to push your physiological systems to the limit without feeling the muscular bloat, heaviness, and exhaustion of such sprints on land.

You can work on technique by performing the same moves in water that you make on land. Of course, the moves will be slower because of water's resistance, but they will be effective nonetheless, for these extra seconds per move allow you to feel your body parts in "freeze frame," which in turn gives you more time for feedback to correct the

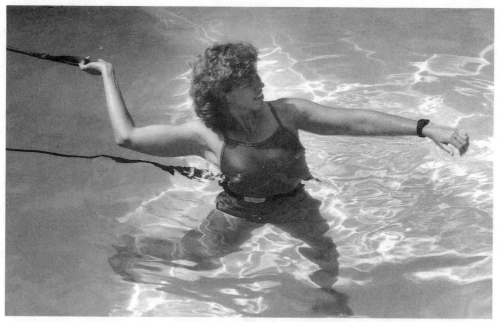

Three-time Olympic javelin thrower Kate Schmidt uses the resistance of tethers and water to practice her form. Some javelin throwers now wear a weight belt and use scuba gear to practice the throw underwater for maximum water resistance.

motions. If you have a coach, the coach's eye also has more time to find any error in the movement that is normally hidden at high speed on land.

In water, you can teach your body to assume your sport's key positions that are difficult to reach on land. For instance, if it's hard for you to bend low enough when putting the shot or hitting a kill shot in racquetball, practice the perfect form in the buoyancy of water until your body learns the "feel" of the correct position. You'll be able to do more repetitions in water without overstressing your knees, and you'll add grace to your movement.

Your Sport-Specific Waterpower Program

Find your sport in the list below. You will see the required fitness **demands** and the **primary muscles** you must strengthen. The **water-training emphasis** is the recommended Waterpower program to perform and the level you should achieve in order to experience success in your sport. Don't start at that level; work your way toward it as set forth in chapters 2 and 3. If you experience pain while attempting The Waterpower Workout, move your training session to deep water and The Deep Waterpower Workout.

To perform the extra sets of the recommended exercises, wait until you've completed your entire program, then perform an additional set of each exercise specified. If you

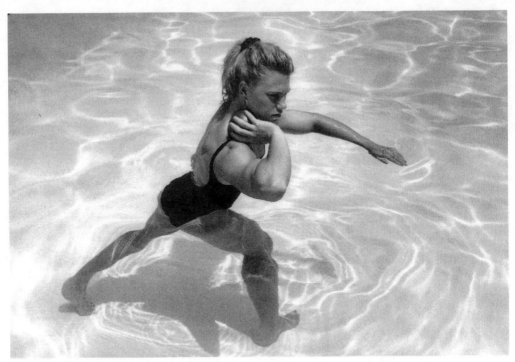

Heptathlete Gea Johnson practices her key position in the shot put.

wish to add two extra sets, go through the list once, then repeat. At the end of each Waterpower or Deep Waterpower Workout session, devote five to ten minutes to your sport-specific skill drills.

As you practice the exercises pertinent to your sport, try to simulate as closely as possible the moves you ordinarily make on land. **The more closely you duplicate the exact skill of your sport, the better your work will transfer back to land.**

The
Complete
Waterpower
Workout
Book

158

BASEBALL

Bo Jackson excelled in both professional football and baseball. After he injured his hip playing football, he refocused his athletic drive on baseball. Chicago White Sox trainer Herm Schneider believed in water therapy and had a SwimEx built into the hydrotherapy room so Bo could perform short, tethered sprints in water. Bo used the Waterpower Workout speed program to help boost his diminished quickness.

Demands: Skill, speed, strength, power, anaerobic capacity, flexibility

Primary muscles: Abdominals, hip flexors, quads, hamstrings, gluteals, rotator cuff, pecs, lats, deltoids, trapezius, teres major, wrist flexors and extensors, biceps, gastroc/soleus complex

Water-training emphasis: The Waterpower Workout, Level 2.
Extra sets of:
Leg Swings (Exercise 11, page 46)
V Kicks (Exercise 8, page 43)
Front/Back Pull (Exercise 26, page 62) adding either Hydro-Tone bells or Speedo SwimMitts (see page 231)

Intervals are eight to ten reps of all-out speed for ten seconds, seven seconds, and five seconds. Count arm strokes to measure speed improvement. Start with thirty- to forty-second recovery periods, and as your anaerobic fitness improves, shorten the recovery time to ten to twenty seconds. See pages 183 and 185 for more details on counting arm strokes.

Exercise 1. Practice Baseball Swing

With an old baseball bat, take twenty to fifty practice swings in chest-deep water. (See Photo 1) Then take the same number of practice swings switch-hitting. In this way, you will strengthen muscles evenly on both sides of your body. Try bunting.

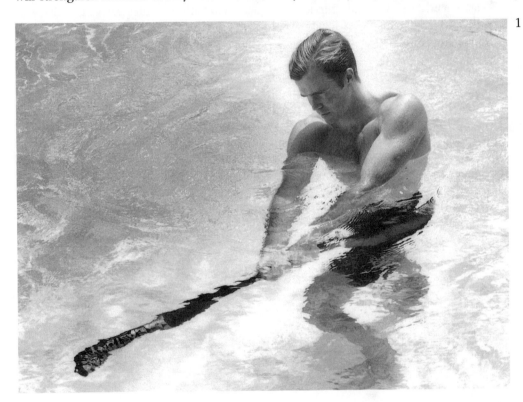

1

The
Complete
Waterpower
Workout
Book

160

BASKETBALL

Demands: Skill, aerobic capacity, speed, power, anaerobic capacity, strength, musculo-skeletal resiliency, flexibility

Primary muscles: Abdominals, hip flexors, gluteals, quads, hamstrings, adductors, gastroc/soleus complex, deltoids, trapezius, pecs, lats

Water-training emphasis: The Twenty-five-Minute Powerhouse Workout (page 78) or Waterpower, Level 3.

Extra sets of:

Power Frog Jumps (Exercise 14, page 49)

Squat Jumps (Exercise 3, page 38)

Side-Straddle Jumps (Exercise 5, page 40)

Front-Straddle Jumps (Exercise 7, page 42)

Use intervals of ten seconds to two minutes with only brief recovery periods between runs.

Exercise 2. Jump Shot

If a sore ankle, knee, or hip won't permit jumping on land, you can retain your timing and jumping ability with this exercise. If you have pain on impact, add a flotation belt to further cushion your landing. If even that slight impact causes pain, skip this exercise and perform Exercise 3 instead.

Find a training partner and an old basketball to take to the pool. Perform your normal jump shot, jumping as high as you can each time. Shoot toward your partner (Photo 2). When the ball is returned, jump high and shoot again. Repeat twenty-five times. (You might be able to persuade your pool director to install a basketball backboard.)

2

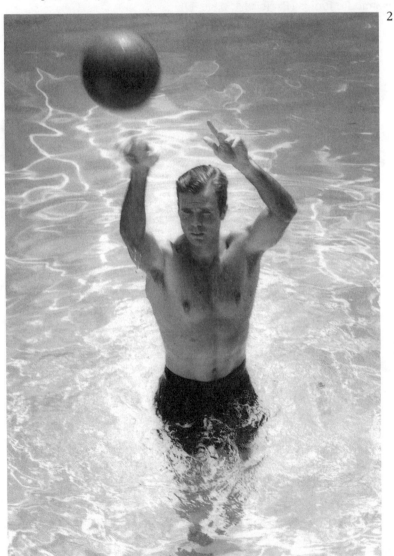

The
Complete
Waterpower
Workout
Book

162

Exercise 3. Deep-Water Jump Shot

Substitute this version of a jump shot if Exercise 2 causes you any pain. Balance on a kick board, a Water Wafer, or an Instructional Swim Barbell as in Photo 3 (see pages 230, 231, and 234 for descriptions of this equipment). Try bending your knees to your chest, then lowering them several times to loosen up the hips, knees, and ankles. If you now have no pain, try performing your jump shot from the kick board, bar, or wafer. First squat, then quickly stand and take your shot before you sink low in the water. Repeat twenty-five times, concentrating on both your shot and your balance.

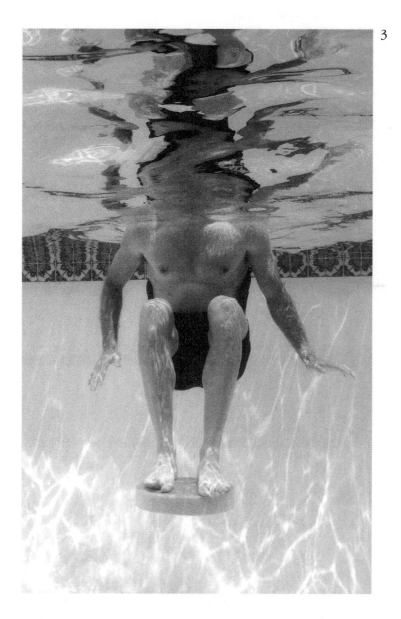

3

CROSS-COUNTRY SKIING

Demands: Aerobic capacity, skill, strength, flexibility

Primary muscles: Gluteus maximus, hip flexors, hamstrings, quads, gastroc/soleus complex, erector spinae, hip adductors and abductors, abdominals, deltoids, lats, pecs, teres major, rhomboids

Water-training emphasis: The Deep Waterpower Workout, Level 3.

Extra sets of:

Intervals (Exercise 8, page 98)

V Kicks (Exercise 11, page 102)

Back Kicks (Exercise 12, page 103)

Straight-Leg Deep Kick (Exercise 19, page 109)

Use intervals of water walking from two minutes to seven minutes in length. Keep recovery periods short. Vary the intensity of your water-walking minutes with speed play. See Exercise 23, this chapter, page 186.

The
Complete
Waterpower
Workout
Book

164

Exercise 4. Cross-Country Stride Practice

In chest-deep water, slide your feet along the bottom of the pool and swing your arms as though cross-country skiing. The harder you work, the more the water will offer counterforce. Use the clock to time your training session to simulate your outdoor workout, since you can't measure distance. Add Speedo SwimMitts (see page 231) to build upper-body power. Add Hydro-Tone boots (see page 231) when you want to work your legs harder (Photo 4).

4

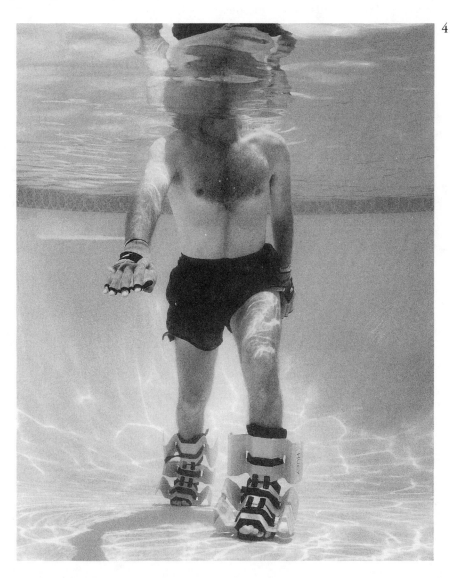

Demands: Aerobic and anaerobic capacity, strength, power, skill

Primary muscles: Quads, gluteus maximus, hamstrings, hip flexors, sartorius, hip adductors, gastroc/soleus complex, pecs, lats, triceps, wrist flexors and extensors

Water-training emphasis: The Deep Waterpower Workout, Level 3.

Extra sets of:

Heel Lifts (Exercise 6, page 96)

Bicycling (Exercise 18, page 108)

Slap Kick (Exercise 21, page 110)

Recreational cyclists use intervals of thirty seconds to two minutes. Competitive cyclists use intervals of ten seconds to five minutes.

Sport-Specific skill drill:

Exercise 5. Deep-Water Cycling

Put on your flotation device and tether yourself to the side of the pool. (See pages 85 and 86 for details.) Maintaining an erect posture, begin a cycling motion with your legs. Unlike deep-water running, your lower leg now circles forward as though making the complete revolution of your bicycle pedals. On the downstroke, point your feet toward the bottom of the pool; on the upstroke, flex your feet toward your head. This plantar (downward) and dorsi (upward) flexion of the foot improves your ankling ability. Substitute this simulated cycling motion for the running motion in all deep-water intervals.

The
Complete
Waterpower
Workout
Book

166

Demands: Musculoskeletal resiliency, strength, power, speed, skill, anaerobic capacity, aerobic capacity, flexibility

Primary muscles: Hip flexors, hamstrings, gluteus maximus, quads, hip adductors and abductors, gastroc/soleus complex, deltoids, pecs, rotator cuffs, trapezius, erector spinae

Water-training emphasis: The Waterpower Workout, Level 2.

Extra sets of:

Lunges (Exercise 1, page 36)

Crossovers (Exercise 2, page 37)

Squat Jumps (Exercise 3, page 38)

Side-Straddle Jumps (Exercise 5, page 40)

Use short, high-intensity sprints for the intervals: five seconds, seven seconds, ten seconds, and twenty seconds. This work requires longer recovery periods, usually two or three times the length of the work period.

Sport-Specific skill drills:

Exercise 6. Catch

Practice the hand-eye coordination of catching an old football while you're in the pool. You must work harder than you would on land to move quickly through the dense water to reach the ball. Sharpen your concentration so that you don't drop the slippery ball once you've caught it. This exercise is good mental and physical practice.

Exercise 7. Run, No Fumble

Tuck the football into your chest. Run back and forth across the pool ten times, maintaining a firm grip on the slippery ball. For variety, you can mix this and the above exercise. First catch the ball, then run across the pool without fumbling.

Exercise 8. Punt/Placekick

Using the resistance of the water instead of an actual ball, practice twenty-five punts or placekicks in the water. Maintain muscle balance by taking twenty-five kicks with your opposite leg.

Sport-Specific
Waterpower
Workouts

GOLF

Demands: Skill, flexibility, strength, power

Primary muscles: Abdominal obliques, hip adductors and abductors, quads, hamstrings, deltoids, lats, teres major, rotator cuffs, triceps, wrist flexors and extensors

Water-training emphasis: The Waterpower or Deep Waterpower Workout, Level 1.

Focus on stretches:

Curl and Stretch (Exercise 27, page 116)

Triangle (Exercise 30, page 66)

Quad Stretch (Exercise 36, page 114)

Hamstring Stretch (Exercise 37, page 115)

Body Swing (Exercise 38, page 117)

Use the basic intervals suggested in chapters 2 and 3.

The
Complete
Waterpower
Workout
Book

168

Exercise 9. Golf Swing

Using the Swing Trainer aqua golf club shown in Photo 9, assume your proper stance in chest-deep water. Step through the motion of your swing, monitoring for any erratic movements. Repeat ten times. Repeat ten more times in the opposite direction to strengthen and stretch both sides of your body. Symmetrical body strength and flexibility are especially important in unilateral sports such as golf that tend to overuse one side of the body while ignoring the other.

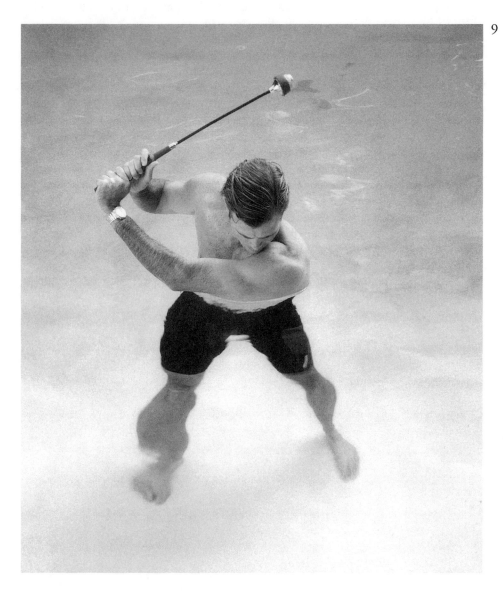

9

**Sport-Specific
Waterpower
Workouts**

GYMNASTICS

Demands: Flexibility, skill, strength, speed, power, musculoskeletal resiliency, anaerobic capacity

Primary muscles: Quads, hamstrings, hip flexors, gluteus maximus, erector spinae, hip adductors and abductors, trapezius, lats, pecs, deltoids, biceps, triceps, wrist flexors and extensors, gastroc/soleus complex

Water-training emphasis: Specialists in parallel bars, uneven parallel bars, rings, pommel horse, and high bar use The Deep Waterpower Workout, Level 3.

Extra sets of:

Waterpower arm exercises (exercises 25 through 29, pages 61 to 65) adding either Hydro-Tone bells or Speedo SwimMitts (see page 231)

Specialists in balance beam and vaulting use The Waterpower Workout, Level 3.

Extra sets of:

Front-Straddle Jumps (Exercise 7, page 42)

V Kicks (Exercise 8, page 43)

Double Heel Lifts (Exercise 9, page 44)

One-Legged Frog Jumps (Exercise 15, page 50)

Specialists in floor exercise use Dance-Specific Waterpower Workouts (Chapter 4).

Extra sets of:

Fourth-Position Extended Barre Stretch (Exercise 5, page 128)

Second-Position Extended Barre Stretch (Exercise 6, page 129)

Grand Rond de Jambe en L'Air (Exercise 13, page 135)

Fondu Developpé Relevé (Exercise 14, page 136)

Battements (Exercise 15, page 137)

Echappés (Exercise 16, page 139)

Cecchetti Pas de Chat (Exercise 19, page 142)

Intervals for all gymnasts should equal the length of time of their event. Vaulters do short, fast sprints; floor exercise performers do intervals as long as their program.

The
Complete
Waterpower
Workout
Book

170

Exercise 10. Balance Beam Practice

Put on some goggles and place dark tape the width of the balance beam on the bottom of the pool. Practice the upright movements of your balance beam routine in waist-deep water. Concentrate on timing, balance, and coordination. The movements will be slowed by water's resistance, so you will gain strength in all of your moves, yet water's buoyancy cushions all of your landings.

Exercise 11. Water Pommel Horse

If you have your own pool and an old pommel horse, put it into the pool so the handles are one to two feet underwater. When grasping the handles, your elbows should be near the surface of the water. Practice your routine. The water's buoyancy lets you teach your body any key positions that trouble you in normal gravity. The resistance you encounter slows your moves and strengthens the primary muscle movers.

Whenever you try new equipment such as the Aquarius Water Workout Station in exercises 12 and 13, it is wise to seek expert supervision. In this way you learn correct form and don't develop bad habits.

Exercise 12. Double Leg Lifts on Aquarius

Face the center of the pool, grasp the top handles, and let your legs dangle straight down. Lift both legs quickly and powerfully toward the surface of the water, then up to the position shown in Photo 12 or higher. Return to the starting position. Perform ten reps.

12

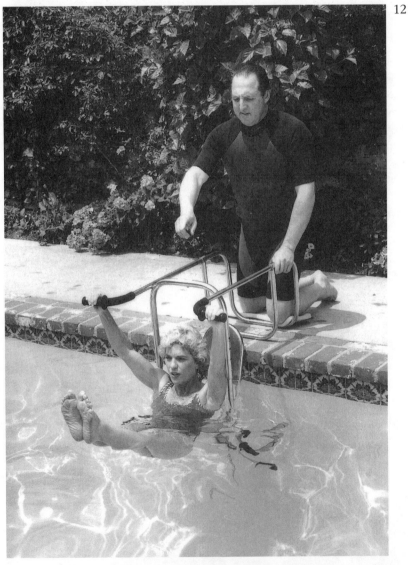

The
Complete
Waterpower
Workout
Book

172

Dr. Dan Silver teaches correct form on the Aquarius.

Exercise 13. Double Side Leg Lifts on Aquarius

Grasp a bottom handle with your left hand and a top handle with your right hand with your legs extending straight down. Swing both legs as far as you can to the right (Photo 13). Return to the starting position. Repeat ten times, then turn and do ten reps facing the other direction.

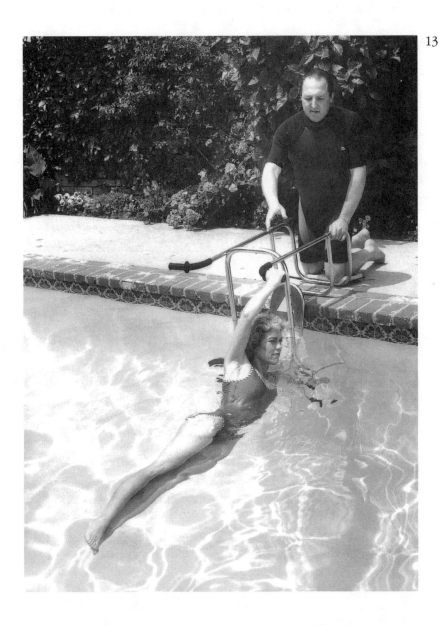

13

Only six weeks prior to the USA Olympic Track and Field Trials, long jumper Mike Powell had an emergency appendectomy. Staples still held his abdomen together, but with his doctor's permission he began The Waterpower Workout classes. He wore flotation devices to decrease his impact upon landing as he performed all the Waterpower exercises. After the class, he worked on his in-air jumping motion and further strengthened his take-off leg with repeated hitch-kick practice. That exercise evolved into Waterpower's one-legged frog jumps.

Demands: Speed, power, musculoskeletal resiliency, strength, skill, flexibility, anaerobic capacity

Primary muscles: Hip flexors, gluteus maximus, quads, hamstrings, gastroc/soleus complex, pecs, deltoids, rhomboids, teres major, trapezius, abdominals, lats, erector spinae, hip adductors

Water-training emphasis: The Twenty-five-Minute Powerhouse Workout (see page 78) or Waterpower Workout, Level 3.

Extra sets of:
Side-Straddle Jumps (Exercise 5, page 40)
Front-Straddle Jumps (Exercise 7, page 42)
Leg Swings (Exercise 11, page 46)
Back Kicks (Exercise 13, page 48)
Power Frog Jumps (Exercise 14, page 49)
Bicycling (Exercise 19, page 56)

Intervals are short, fast sprints from ten to thirty seconds with equal or double recovery time.

Sport-Specific skill drills:

Exercise 14. One-Legged Frog Jumps *(Exercise 15, page 50)*

Perform the basic exercise until you are comfortable with the coordination, then add the arm movements applicable to your jump. Perform thirty to forty reps with one leg, then thirty to forty reps with the other leg.

The
Complete
Waterpower
Workout
Book

174

Exercise 15. In-Air Practice

Stand at the end of the diving board farthest from the pool. Take several quick strides, then drive powerfully up and off the board using your usual take-off leg. Practice your normal in-air movement patterns for the long jump—hitch kick or sail—then land in the water. You will have more air time in which to learn or perfect your in-air movements. If your pool has no diving board, run and jump off the side as Gea Johnson does in Photo 15.

15

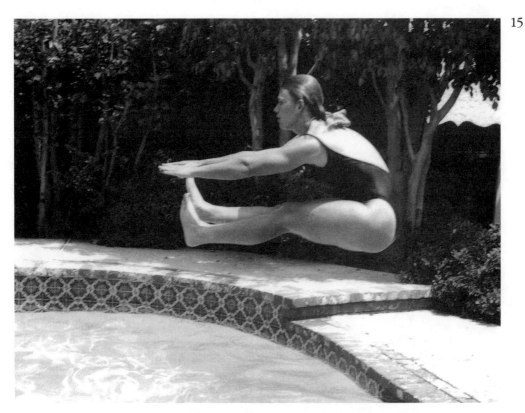

Triple jumper Al Joyner came to The Waterpower Workout class with a wooden boot on his broken foot. He and the boot went straight into the water and he completed the entire workout without pain. He simulated his bounds in chest-deep water to keep his powerful technique fresh. A few months later, Al won a gold medal in the 1984 Los Angeles Olympic Games.

Exercise 16. Bounds

Bounding is a technique all jumpers must master. Stand on both feet with your weight evenly distributed between them. Simultaneously drive your left knee forward and up and your bent right arm up to the position shown in Photo 16. You must push forcefully with your right leg and foot to gain height away from the pool bottom. Once you have pushed off, **keep your push-off leg straight** and strive for as much "hangtime" in this position as possible. When your left foot touches down, immediately push off into the next bound with your right knee and left arm forward. Perform twenty to forty bounds. Gently kick out your legs to relax them. Repeat.

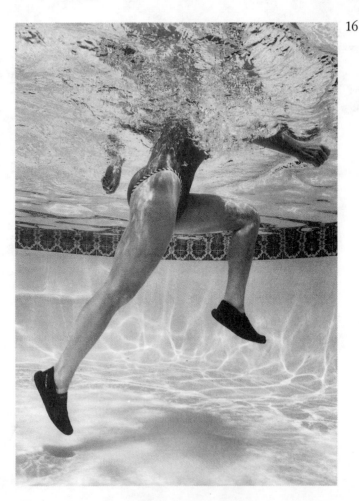

16

The
Complete
Waterpower
Workout
Book

176

Exercise 17. High Jump Approach and Takeoff

In waist-deep water, step off the strides of your high jump approach. These measurements aren't likely to be the same as on land because of the water resistance. Your movements will be slowed by that resistance, so as you perform each repetition, focus on your balance, foot placement, and the precise body angle you must assume at takeoff.

MARTIAL ARTS

Actress Cybill Shepherd experienced chondromalacia (pain behind the kneecap) a month prior to the shooting of her karate movie Stormy Weathers. *Because she couldn't train on land, she did The Deep Waterpower Workout, then performed ten front kicks, ten side kicks, and ten back kicks with each leg.*

Demands: Skill, strength, power, flexibility, speed, musculoskeletal resiliency, anaerobic capacity

Primary muscles: Quads, hamstrings, hip flexors, gluteus maximus, erector spinae, hip abductors and adductors, gastroc/soleus complex, pecs, deltoids, rhomboids, trapezius, teres major

Water-training emphasis: The Waterpower Workout or Deep Waterpower Workout, Level 3.

Extra sets of the following if you are using The Waterpower Workout:

    Leg Swings (Exercise 11, page 46)
    Back Kicks (Exercise 13, page 48)
    Scissors (Exercise 21, page 58)

Extra sets of the following if you are using The Deep Waterpower Workout:

    Flies (Exercise 10, page 101)
    V Kicks (Exercise 11, page 102)
    Back Kicks (Exercise 12, page 103)
    Scissors (Exercise 22, page 111)

Intervals are primarily short fast sprints, but occasionally include a one- to two-minute hard run or forceful power walk.

Sport-Specific skill drills:

Exercise 18. Karate Kick

Using your most precise form and appropriate breathing pattern, practice twenty to forty front kicks with your right leg. Repeat with the left leg. Perform the same number of side kicks (right and left), then back kicks (right and left).

18A

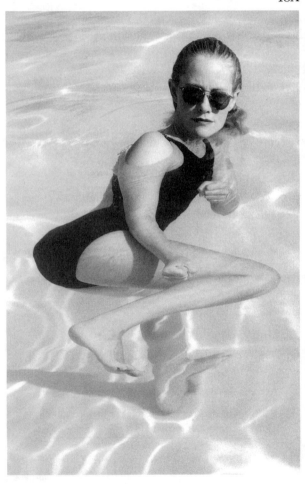

18B

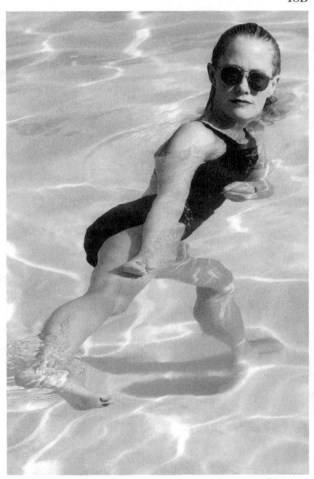

Exercise 19. Karate Punch

Concentrate on explosive power as you perform twenty to forty punches to the front with each arm (Photos 19A, 19B). Then practice the same number of punches to the side with each arm. Add resistance equipment for additional strength gains.

19A

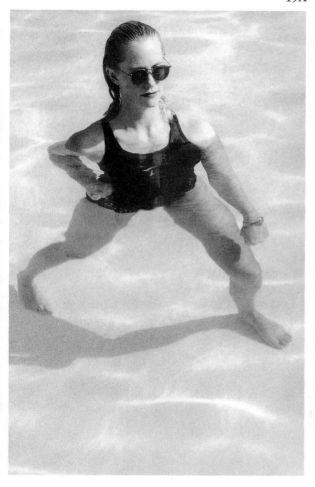

19B

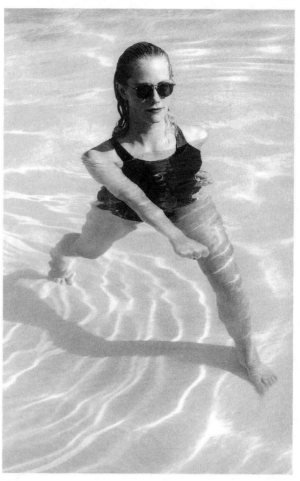

RACKET SPORTS

John Lloyd plays professional tennis for the Los Angeles Strings and in the over-thirty-five category of the Grand Champions. In 1990, he was ranked number one in the world even though he suffered from a strained right hamstring most of the year and did virtually all of his running and conditioning in the pool.

Of all the Waterpower Workout exercises, John found the sprints on a tether (Exercise 22, page 184) and Knee Jumps (Exercise 21, page 182) most valuable. Although John previously did similar jumps on land to strengthen the muscles needed for overhead smashes, he now jumps primarily in water to avoid impact on landing.

Demands: Skill, strength, speed, power, aerobic capacity, anaerobic capacity, flexibility, musculoskeletal resiliency

Primary muscles: Quads, hamstrings, gastroc/soleus complex, hip flexors, gluteus maximus, abdominals, abdominal obliques, pecs, deltoids, trapezius, rhomboids, teres major, wrist flexors and extensors, hip adductors and abductors

Water-training emphasis: The Twenty-five-Minute Powerhouse Workout or Waterpower Workout, Level 3.

Extra sets of:

Back Kicks (Exercise 13, page 48)

Power Frog Jumps (Exercise 14, page 49)

One-Legged Frog Jumps (Exercise 15, page 50)

Arm exercises (Exercises 25 through 29, pages 61 to 65) adding Hydro-Tone bells or Speedo SwimMitts (see page 231).

Use a variety of intervals from ten seconds to three minutes. Sample intervals workout:

Four × ten seconds, recover twenty seconds between each

Two × thirty seconds, recover thirty seconds between each

Two × one minute, recover forty-five seconds between each

One × three minutes, recover forty-five seconds afterward

Keep the recovery time short, the equivalent of time between points played on the court.

The
Complete
Waterpower
Workout
Book

180

Exercise 20. Racket Swing

Choose your oldest racket to take into the water. Walk through the exact motion of your forehand twenty-five times (Photo 20). Because the water slows you down, you have the opportunity to feel each segment of your stroke and work on any weak or awkward spot. Next, turn and step into twenty-five backhand strokes, concentrating on form.

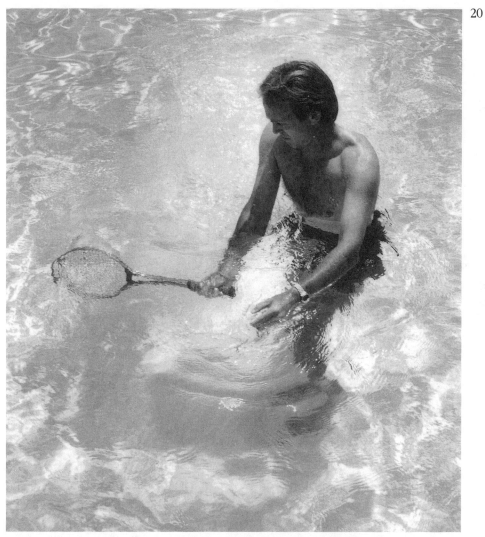

20

Change hands and work the opposite side to prevent body imbalances that come from unilateral sports. Do twenty-five forehands and twenty-five backhands with your nondominant hand.

Exercise 21. Knee Jumps

Bounce on both feet with your arms reaching straight overhead. Hold your arms steady as you jump and lift both knees toward your chest (Photo 21). When your feet return to the pool bottom, push off and immediately lift both knees again.

21

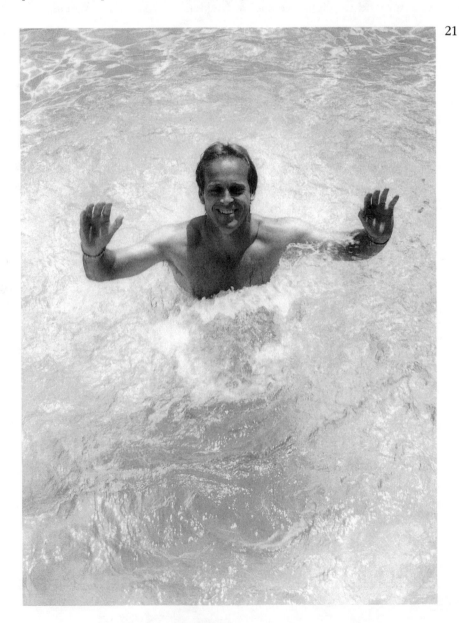

The
Complete
Waterpower
Workout
Book

182

RUNNING AND SPRINTING

If a foot, ankle, leg, hip, or back injury keeps you from running in shallow water, skip exercises 22 and 23 and move directly to deep water in Exercise 24.

Regardless of the depth of the water, a tether is a necessary ingredient. It lets the sprinter achieve the proper lean; it helps distance runners and others lock themselves into good body alignment; it holds all athletes in place. Whenever a runner's form is suspect in the water, add a tether. (See page 86.)

Florence Griffith Joyner suffered a hamstring strain that prevented her from running at top speed on land, so her coach Bobby Kersee brought her to The Waterpower Workout for sprint training. An elasticized tether attached between her waist and a ladder held her in the forward-lean position of the sprinter. She retained her flawless arm action and high knee lift as she ran in place. Then she actually increased her sprint speed by working forcefully against the water's resistance: She counted arm strokes for ten-second sprints. At first she performed twenty-five right/left arm strokes (she counted "one" each time her right hand pushed forward). Over the next two weeks she improved that turnover rate to thirty-four arm strokes in ten seconds. Months later, in the 1988 Seoul Olympics, she won three gold medals and one silver. (Florence's sister-in-law Jackie Joyner-Kersee demonstrates in Photo 22.)

Demands: Speed, strength, power, anaerobic capacity, flexibility, musculoskeletal resiliency, skill, aerobic capacity

Primary muscles: Hamstrings, quads, gluteus maximus, hip flexors, gastroc/soleus complex, hip adductors, pecs, deltoids, trapezius, rhomboids, teres major, bicep, tricep

Water-training emphasis: The Twenty-five-Minute Powerhouse Workout or Waterpower Workout, Level 3. If you have a weight-bearing injury, do The Deep Waterpower Workout, Level 3, until you can gradually move to shallow water.

Extra sets of the following if you are using the Waterpower Workout:
Side-Straddle Jumps (Exercise 5, page 40)
Single Heel Lifts (Exercise 6, page 41)
Double Heel Lifts (Exercise 9, page 44)
Leg Swings (Exercise 11, page 46)
Back Kicks (Exercise 13, page 48)
Bicycling (Exercise 19, page 56)

Extra sets of the following if you are using the Deep Waterpower Workout:
Flies (Exercise 10, page 101)
V-Kicks (Exercise 11, page 102)
Abdominals (Exercise 9, page 100)
Back Kicks (Exercise 12, page 103)

Intervals should approximate the length of time you run on land. Sprinters use ten second to ninety second intervals. Distance runners use two minute to ten minute intervals. Marathoners can deep-water run for up to two hours or more.

Sport-Specific
Waterpower
Workouts

Exercise 22. Sprint on a Tether

Strap on the waistband of a Waterpower Workout Tether or a Perry Band (see page 86). Begin running in place in waist- to chest-deep water, concentrating on good sprint form: The head and chest are erect, the shoulders are down and stable, eyes look straight ahead. Your hands should break the surface of the water. The knees lift to 90 degrees while the arms pull directly forward and back—no lateral movement. Opposition is vital. Be sure the opposite arm and leg work together. The angle of the arm at the elbow remains the same throughout the motion. There is movement only at the shoulder, not at the wrist or elbow.

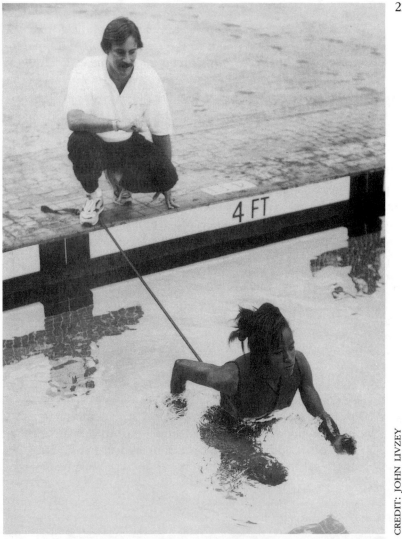

22

The
Complete
Waterpower
Workout
Book

184

CREDIT: JOHN LIVZEY

Robert Forster, P.T., assists three-time Olympic gold medalist Jackie Joyner-Kersee with interval training on a tether.

As soon as good running form has been established, begin increasing the pace. Try running at a slow, medium, and fast pace while maintaining good form. Then try sprinting in water. If your form crumbles, begin again at a slow pace and work your way back up to a sprint. If your feet slip on the bottom of the pool, or if you feel blisters forming on your toes, put on a pair of water-training shoes (Photo 16, page 176).

Plan your interval training based on the work you would do if you were on the track. Instead of measuring workouts by distance, however, measure them by time. For instance, if you planned to run four × 400-meter intervals in approximately sixty seconds each, do the same work while sprinting on the tether: Sprint at the same level of effort it would take you to run the imaginary 400 meters and continue for sixty seconds. A training partner with a stopwatch or a large poolside clock can help you time the work accurately. Lightly jog for your rest period between intervals. Your leg muscles won't feel "pumped up," so you won't require as much rest time as you would normally on the track.

Running speed is stride length times stride frequency. Because sprinters run powerfully *in place* in the water, the only way to measure speed is by counting arm strokes, which correspond to stride frequency. Run for sixty seconds at a comfortable pace, counting each time your right arm swings forward. Give yourself a thirty- to forty-five-second recovery jog, then run sixty seconds again, trying to beat that number. Now that you know how much effort it takes and at what point in the minute you become tired, try to beat that number again. Start fast and keep your concentration tightly locked on your rhythm and form, especially when you approach your fatigue zone. Try counting arm strokes for forty-five-second intervals, thirty-second intervals, and ten-second sprints. Keep a record of your best scores as a measurement of speed improvement.

Once you've mastered a Waterpower sprint session, add the psychological component for an even better workout. Choose a favorite track in your mind and visualize yourself moving around the track as you run. For instance, as you run the first fifteen seconds of your 400 meters, picture yourself moving around the first turn. Between fifteen and thirty seconds, imagine the sensation of striding down the backstretch. From thirty to forty-five seconds you run around the second turn, then in the final fifteen seconds, increase velocity as you drive down the homestretch to the finish line. By adding this vital aspect of the workout, you retain confidence in your fitness and racing capability. A coach or training partner can talk you through the interval, even spicing it up with a commentary that includes your rivals.

If you wish to do this interval training, but don't know your approximate time for distances on a track, use this basic equation, which is easy to see and compute on a clock or stopwatch.

50 meters = 7 seconds	300 meters = 45 seconds
100 meters = 15 seconds	400 meters = 60 seconds
200 meters = 30 seconds	800 meters = 2 minutes

(Although you can simply transfer your track workout to the pool, you may wish to actually increase the work load. Because you do no pounding, and because the hamstrings and gluteals don't "tie up" from fatigue, you can perform more sprints in the water than on land. Try adding one more long sprint than normal or two extra short sprints. Long sprints are 300 to 600 meters and short sprints are 50 to 200 meters.)

Exercise 23. Distance Running on a Tether

Tether yourself to the side of the pool. Even though you run the mile, 3,000-meter, 5-kilometer, 10-kilometer, half-marathon, and marathon races, you will also do workouts in water based on time rather than distance.

Begin running slowly in place, focusing on good form. Gradually increase your speed until you have reached the exertion level of your usual "training pace" used on distance runs. Sustain that effort for five to thirty minutes, depending on your race. The shorter the race, the shorter the steady-paced warm-up run.

Distance runners tend to overlook the importance of stretching, so spend at least five minutes doing the stretching exercises (Exercise 30, page 66, exercises 36 through 38, pages 73 to 75, and Exercise 27, page 116) before moving on to your interval training.

Then duplicate one of your land-based workouts in the pool. Simply use time instead of distance as your measuring device. Provide ample recovery time between intervals so that the quality of your running doesn't diminish. If you don't have an established interval training routine, try adding variety to your distance work with *fartlek,* the Swedish word for speed play. Run one fast minute, one easy minute, then one moderate minute. Continue for ten to fifteen minutes choosing a variety of speeds, changing each minute.

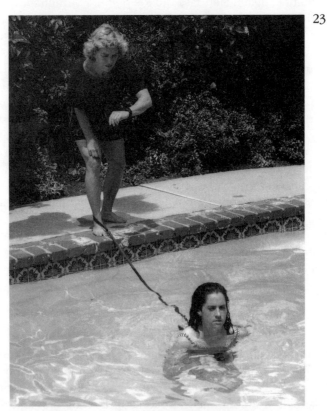

23

The
Complete
Waterpower
Workout
Book

186

Lynda Huey coaches distance runner Laurie Chapman.

Exercise 24. Deep-Water Sprints or Distance Running

Put on a flotation device and tether yourself to the side of the deep end of the pool. Duplicate the good running form you use on land. See page 88 for details of deep-water running form. Perform the same intervals discussed in the previous exercises, 22 and 23, but here without touching the bottom of the pool.

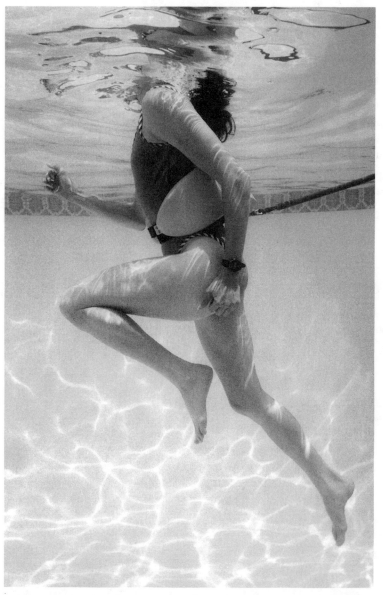

24

Distance running on a tether can be performed with the feet touching the pool bottom or while suspended.

Demands: Skill, speed, aerobic capacity, strength, power, musculoskeletal resiliency, flexibility, anaerobic capacity

Primary muscles: Hip flexors, quads, hamstrings, gluteus maximus, gastroc/soleus complex, hip adductors and abductors, trapezius, lats, pecs, rhomboids, teres major, biceps, triceps, scalenes, sternocleidomastoids, abdominals, abdominal obliques, tibialis anterior

Water-training emphasis: The Twenty-five-Minute Powerhouse Workout or Waterpower Workout, Level 3.

Extra sets of:

Side-Straddle Jumps (Exercise 5, page 40)

Double Heel Lifts (Exercise 9, page 44)

Leg Swings (Exercise 11, page 46)

One-Legged Frog Jumps (Exercise 15, page 50)

Slap Kicks (Exercise 24, page 60)

Intervals range from ten-second sprints to five-minute buildup runs (each minute gets faster).

Sport-Specific skill drill:

Exercise 25. Soccer Practice

Without a ball, practice the action of kicking the soccer ball with first one foot and then the other. Duplicate any of the agility drills you perform on land in the pool. Gain strength and speed by moving quickly against water's resistance.

The
Complete
Waterpower
Workout
Book

188

VOLLEYBALL

Demands: Skill, strength, speed, power, musculoskeletal resiliency, aerobic capacity, anaerobic capacity

Primary muscles: Deltoids, pecs, wrist flexors and extensors, abdominals, abdominal obliques, rhomboids, lats, teres major, quads, gluteus maximus, hamstrings, gastroc/soleus complex, hip flexors, hip adductors and abductors

Water-training emphasis: The Twenty-five-Minute Powerhouse Workout or Waterpower Workout, Level 3.

Extra sets of:

Crossovers (Exercise 2, page 37)

Squat Jumps (Exercise 3, page 38)

Double Heel Lifts (Exercise 9, page 44)

Power Frog Jumps (Exercise 14, page 49)

One-Legged Frog Jumps (Exercise 15, page 50)

Intervals focus primarily on short sprints, but include an occasional two-minute buildup run (each minute gets faster).

Exercise 26. Jump and Block

Coaching partner: Spike an old volleyball toward your partner. Vary the speed of your hits. Your partner will time his or her jumps and blocks accordingly.

Working partner: React quickly to each spiked ball that is hit toward you. Jump high (Photo 26), blocking the ball into the water. Watch the ball until you've made contact with it. Toss the ball back to your partner and prepare for the next block.

26

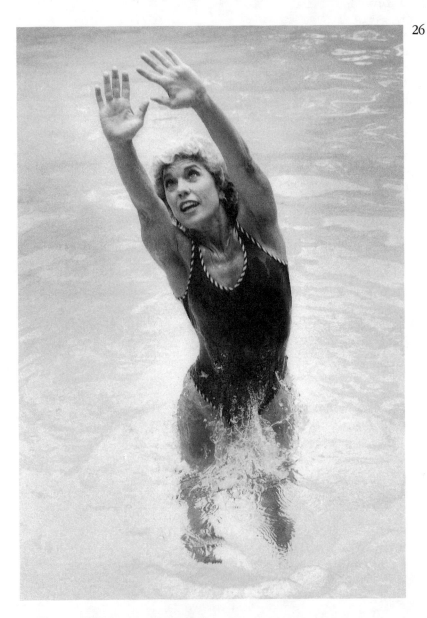

The
Complete
Waterpower
Workout
Book

190

Exercise 27. Digging Practice

Coaching partner: Spike an imaginary ball either to the right or to the left of your partner's feet. Vary the order of your pantomimed spikes from right to left so that your partner has to think and react.

Working partner: React quickly to each spiking motion, bending the appropriate knee and swinging both arms into proper placement for a solid dig (Photo 27).

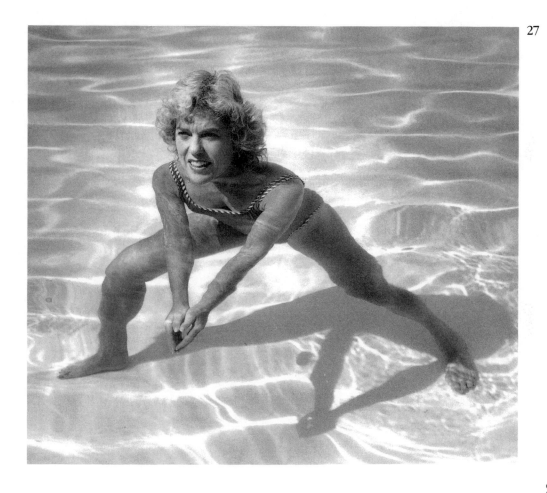

27

Sport-Specific Circuit Training

Sports competition requires physical as well as mental agility—the ability to move from one place to another quickly and to perform a designated skill. The following example of a circuit specific to tennis should give you ideas for setting up one for your sport.

After a warm-up, perform each of these circuit exercises for two minutes. **Rest one minute between exercises** as you move between stations in the circuit.

SHALLOW CIRCUIT (CHEST-DEEP WATER)

Exercise 1. Sprint on a Tether

In shallow water, tether yourself to the side of the pool. Run easily for fifteen seconds, then sprint fifteen seconds. Alternate easy running and sprinting every fifteen seconds until you have completed the two-minute period. Remove the tether and move to the second station, where an old tennis racket is waiting for you poolside.

Exercise 2. Racket Swing

Perform forehand strokes in the water for one minute with your dominant arm, then switch to your nondominant arm for the second minute. Replace the racket on the side of the pool and pick up two Hydro-Tone bells at the third station.

The
Complete
Waterpower
Workout
Book

192

Exercise 3. Hydro-Tone Bicep/Tricep Curl

Hydro-Tone equipment offers three-dimensional resistance to the water to provide you with the equivalent of a weight-training workout. Stabilize your arms by resting your upper arms and elbows against the side of the pool (Photo C). Your elbows remain in contact with the pool wall as you pull your hands toward your chest (Photo D), then push them back to the starting position. Use equal speed and force in both halves of this exercise (the pull and the push phases) to retain muscle balance. Continue for two minutes. Then place the bells poolside and move to station four.

C

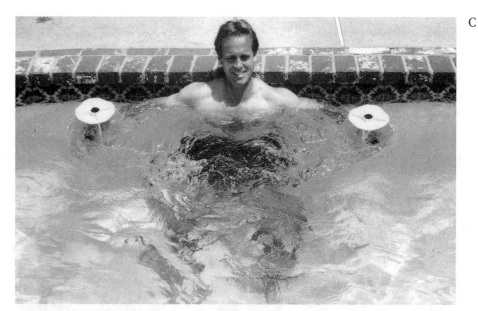

D

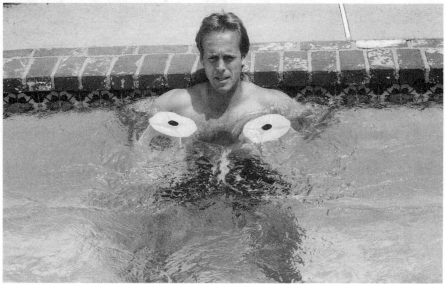

Exercise 4. Knee Jumps

Holding your hands overhead, jump and lift both knees to your chest (Photo 21, p. 182). When your feet touch the bottom of the pool, jump again. Keep this up for two minutes. Move to station five, where you will find Hydro-Tone Boots on the side of the pool.

Exercise 5. Hydro-Tone Hamstring Curl

Pull a Hydro-Tone boot onto your left foot and using the form shown in photos E and F, perform hamstring curls for one minute. (See Exercise 35, page 72, for the basic exercise, but use the modifications shown in the photos to gain best advantage from the equipment.) Don't let your knee move forward or backward. Knee stability lets you isolate the hamstring muscle. After one minute, switch the boot to your right foot and continue for the second minute.

E
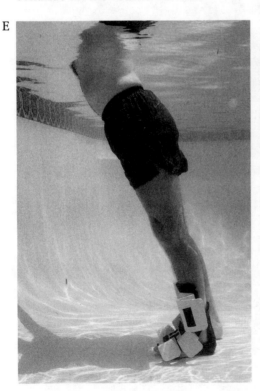
F
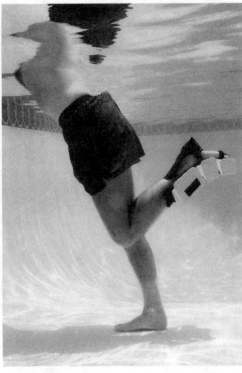

The
Complete
Waterpower
Workout
Book

194

You have now completed the circuit for the first time. Stretch for two to three minutes, then repeat the circuit.

Notice that the sport-specific exercises are 2 and 4. The other exercises strengthen muscle groups important to tennis. If you can think of only one exercise specific to your sport, do it at the number two position and repeat it in the fourth position.

Put on a flotation device (see pages 85 and 86) and at each station in the circuit perform the appropriate exercise for two minutes. Rest one minute between stations.

Exercise 1. Power Walk with Speedo SwimMitts XT

Speedo SwimMitts offer increased water resistance as you do your deep-water walking (see Exercise 2, page 90). Pull on a pair and hold your hands wide in the power position (Photo G) for maximum resistance as you water walk for two minutes. Remove the Speedo SwimMitts and pick up the Instructional Swim Barbell on the side of the pool.

G

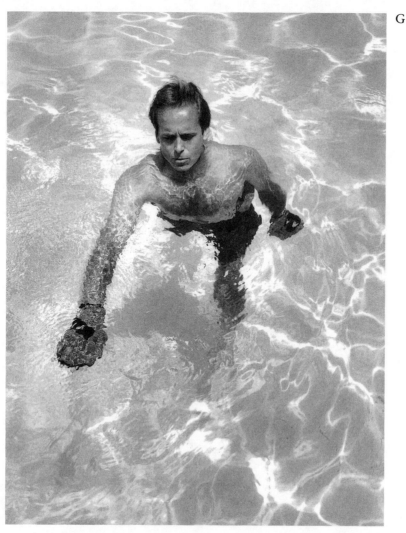

Sport-Specific
Waterpower
Workouts

Exercise 2. Barbell Jump Overs

This requires good lower back and hamstring flexibility. If it is too difficult for you to do now, set yourself a goal of improving your flexibility. If you currently have lower back pain, do not do this exercise.

Grasp the Instructional Swim Barbell with both hands and assume a balanced position as shown in Photo H. Tuck your knees toward your chest and shoot your legs over the bar. Bend your knees again and return to the starting position. Jump back and forth through the bar for two minutes. Place the barbell on the side of the pool, then move at least an arm's distance away from the side of the pool.

H

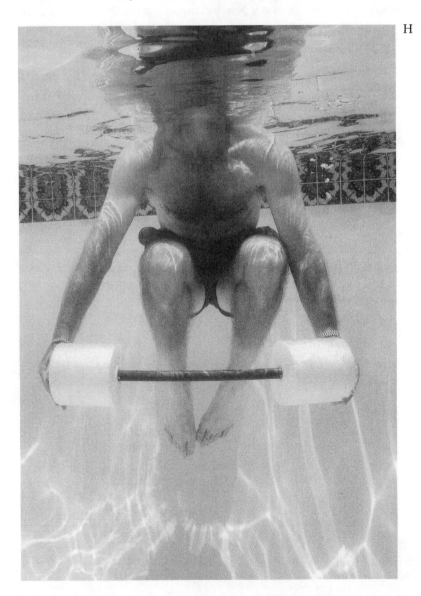

The
Complete
Waterpower
Workout
Book

196

Exercise 3. Abdominals *(Exercise 9, page 100)*

Perform the basic exercise for the first minute, then the variation for the second minute. Next, pick up a kick board, barbell, or Water Wafer from the side of the pool.

Exercise 4. Jump Turns on Water Wafer

Balance on a Water Wafer, a kick board, or an Instructional Swim Bar with your knees bent as in Photo I. Quickly stand up, making a turn to your right, then bending both knees once again to regain your balance. Start with 90-degree turns and work your way up to 180-degree turns. Continue turning to your right for the first minute, then reverse your turns for the second minute. Place the float poolside.

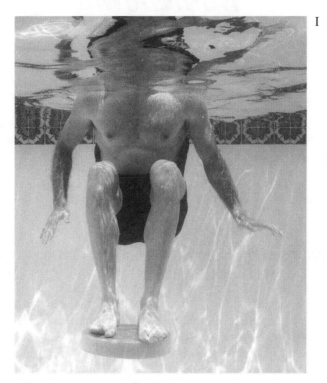

I

Exercise 5. Flies *(Exercise 10, page 101.)*

Work with speed and power at this for two minutes.

This completes the deep-water circuit. After stretching for two to three minutes, repeat the entire circuit. As you become stronger, increase the length of the work period or reduce the length of the recovery period between exercises.

The Waterpower Warm-Down

The demands placed on the body during exercise leave the muscles and the circulatory system in an altered state when exercise is completed. The blood vessels respond to the increased needs of the working muscles and the production of heat during exercise and increase three to five times in diameter in a physiological event known as vasodilation. Thus a greater volume of blood enters the capillary beds housed in and around the muscles. It is here that oxygen and nutrients are delivered to the working muscles and carbon dioxide and other waste products leave the muscle cells and enter the circulatory system.

Although the pumping action of the heart is responsible for blood reaching the muscles, there is no parallel system to return the blood to the heart and lungs for revitalization. Instead, the body relies largely on skeletal muscle contraction to squeeze the blood through the veins back toward the heart. As the muscles of the limbs contract, they exert pressure on the veins in the immediate vicinity, and blood is pushed along its path. Valves housed in the veins allow the blood to flow in one direction only—toward the heart.

The
Complete
Waterpower
Workout
Book

198

When exercise stops abruptly, the muscles are left with large volumes of waste-laden blood without a means for getting home. In the instances where exercise is performed in the upright posture, there is a pooling of blood in the legs. The faster this blood is returned to the heart, as when one performs a warm-down, the faster the body can return to its normal state of functioning called homeostasis.

Lactic acid is a natural by-product of muscle cell metabolism during brief bouts of relatively high intensity exercise. Studies have shown that when an athlete performs rhythmic exercise after workouts, lactic acid is removed from the muscles and blood 50 percent faster than if the athlete comes to an abrupt, complete stop.

Delayed onset muscle soreness (DOMS) is common after high-intensity exercise and occurs most often twenty-four to forty-eight hours after an early-season workout or when the workout intensity is increased abruptly at any time of the year. This soreness has been attributed to several possible causes: muscle cell damage, connective tissue damage, muscle spasm, or swelling that stimulates sensory nerve endings. Although it is not known which of these theories is correct, there is evidence that postworkout stretching decreases or alleviates DOMS. It is also known that after exercise, muscles are left in a shortened and swollen state. By means of stretching and lengthening exercises, the muscles are returned to their normal resting length and are better prepared for total recovery. Furthermore, stretching helps "wring" the edema (swelling) from the fluid-filled muscle tissues. The hydrostatic pressure of water further flushes waste products (the by-products of muscle contraction) out of the muscle tissues into the bloodstream. The massaging effect of movement through water assists the return of blood to the heart.

The Waterpower Warm-Down provides both stretching and rhythmic movements, offering a thorough warm-down at the end of land-based exercise. This warm-down has been used with both elite and recreational athletes and has become invaluable as an integral part of their training programs. (Track coach Randy Huntington insists that Olympic long jumper Mike Powell spend ten to fifteen minutes in the pool after *every* workout.)

Until recently, most athletes simply continued their usual activity for their warm-down. Sprinters jogged slowly around the track; cyclists took a few leisurely turns around the course; swimmers kicked an extra length or two.

But in the past few years, athletes from all sports—basketball, volleyball, football, baseball, track and field, cycling, and more—have learned to use water wisely. They use it not only for cross training or workouts while injured, but they now use it for extended, miraculous warm-downs. Miraculous, because athletes can enter the pool after their normal warm-down *knowing* they will be sore tomorrow and wind up feeling thoroughly freshened, loosened, and relaxed. Even marathoners can avoid the acute soreness that usually follows a race by doing The Waterpower Warm-Down.

The Waterpower Warm-Down is your key to preventing DOMS. Additionally, **it can be the perfect workout for you on a day when you don't feel like doing your usual workout.** You may be tired, sore, or simply not motivated for land-based exercise.

The Waterpower Workout and The Deep Waterpower Workout in chapters 2 and 3 contain their own built-in warm-downs. The two series of exercises below are specifically designed to be self-contained sessions for post-land-based programs or recovery-day workouts by themselves. Choose the **Shallow** program if your muscles are sore, but not your joints. Select the **Deep** program if your joints feel overworked.

Do the twenty-minute Waterpower Warm-Down program:
- Immediately after a land-based workout in which you have overexerted. You will be less sore tomorrow.
- After a sprint workout. "Untie" those knots in your hamstrings and gluteals.
- After a long plane flight. A Waterpower Warm-Down will help alleviate jet lag.
- Following a session of power lifting. The massaging effects of water will ease out much of your soreness and fatigue.
- If you are physically or mentally tired and don't feel up to your normal day's training schedule. You will feel rejuvenated after a Waterpower Warm-Down.

SHALLOW WATERPOWER WARM-DOWN

Although these exercises are similar to their counterparts in The Waterpower Workout, Chapter 2, there are significant differences. Read the instructions and look at the photographs carefully.

Follow these tips for maximum benefit:

- Move slowly.
- Emphasize range of motion instead of power.
- Stretch and loosen the body; don't create more work load.
- Sink low in the water, allowing the water's buoyancy to hold you up rather than making your legs do the work.
- Add a flotation belt if you wish to diminish further the work load on your legs.
- Begin each movement cautiously and slowly. If you encounter soreness, continue moving at a reduced pace while gradually reaching for full range of motion.

Enter the pool and move to upper-chest-deep water. **Do each of the following exercises ten to fifteen times in the order presented. Then repeat the entire sequence, 1 through 8.** Begin Exercise 1 immediately so you will not become cold.

The
Complete
Waterpower
Workout
Book

200

Exercise 1. Lunges

This first exercise lets you become acclimated to the water temperature and begins the warm-down process.

   Start in a lunge position, your left foot a full stride in front of your right foot. Your right arm should be forward for counterbalance (Photo 1). Gently jump up and switch arm and leg positions so that the right leg and left arm are now forward. Emphasize the rhythmic swing of the arms; avoid jumping high. This exercise has two parts, so each right-left cycle should be counted as only one repetition.

1

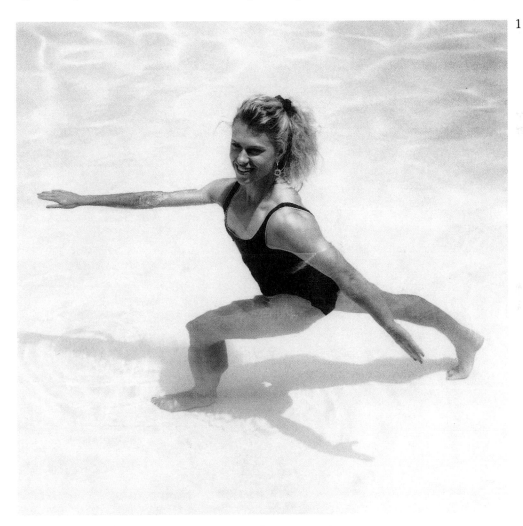

**The Waterpower
Warm-Down**

Exercise 2. Crossovers

If you have any leg or arm soreness, you will feel it and will begin the loosening process during Crossovers. Move gently and slowly.

Begin in a wide-stride position with arms out to your sides as in Photo 2A. Gently jump up and cross the right arm over the left arm and the right leg over the left leg before landing, as in Photo 2B. Jump again to the wide-stride starting position. Now jump and cross the left arm and leg over the right arm and leg. Continue, alternating the arm and leg that are on top. Emphasize balance and control, not height of jump. Crossing and opening is one repetition.

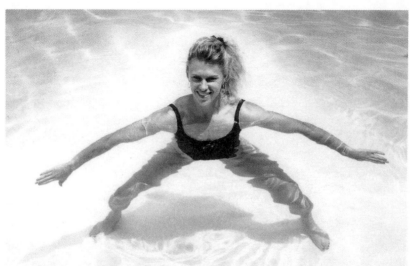

2A

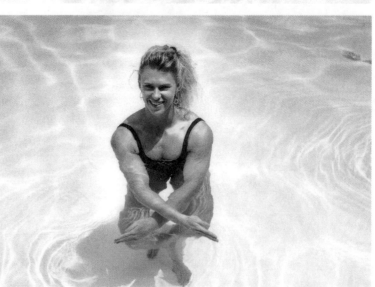

2B

The
Complete
Waterpower
Workout
Book

202

Exercise 3. V Kicks

This exercise eases soreness from adductors, gluteals, and hamstrings.

Stay low in the water as you bounce from one foot to the other, from side to side, lifting one knee, then the other. Lifting the left knee, then the right makes one repetition. After ten to fifteen reps, straighten the legs into V Kicks as shown in Photo 3. Stay low in the water as you do another ten to fifteen reps.

3

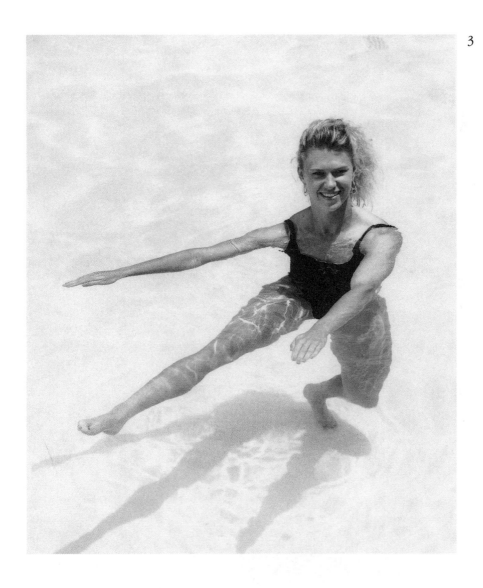

**The Waterpower
Warm-Down**

Exercise 4. Reverse Rocking Horse

This smooth, rhythmic exercise keeps you moving, continuing your warm-down with little effort. The arms assist your body's forward and backward rocking motion in this warm-down version rather than resist the movement in the workout version.

Bounce on your right foot and hold your left leg straight to the front. Extend both arms to the front as in Photo 4A. Sweep both arms back to your sides along the water's surface and bounce forward onto your left foot (Photo 4B). Next, sweep the arms forward to the starting position and bounce back onto your right foot. Rock forward and back ten times, then repeat with reverse foot positions (right foot forward and left foot back) ten more cycles.

4A

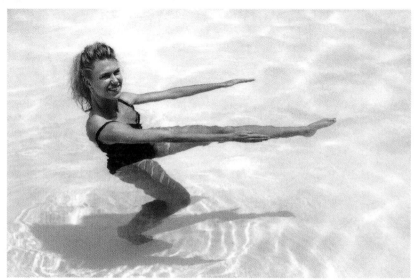

4B

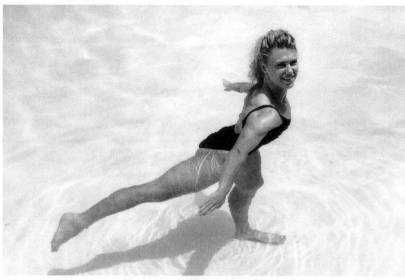

The
Complete
Waterpower
Workout
Book

204

Exercise 5. Front Kicks

Front kicks further stretch and loosen the hamstrings and lower back.

Move to slightly deeper water. Sit low in the water as you lift your right leg in front of you. Bounce on your left foot and reach forward with your left arm for counterbalance (Photo 5). Although the workout version of this requires straight legs, the warm-down version allows you to bend your knees if your hamstrings or lower back is stiff. Jump up easily and switch arm and leg positions so that the left leg is now in front of you and the right arm is forward. A right-left cycle is one repetition. As your muscles loosen, gradually straighten your knees.

5

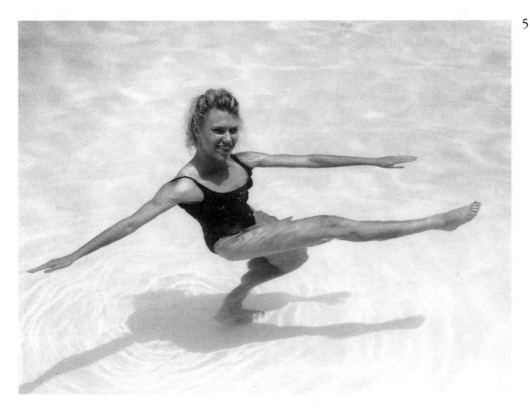

Exercise 6. Back Kicks

This is a key exercise for sprinters, hurdlers, jumpers, and all those who experience "bootie lock," a tying up of the gluteal muscles. If executed within several hours of a maximal-effort workout, it can eliminate DOMS.

Move to shallower water so you can bend forward and not get water in your face or mouth. Stand on your left leg and reach your right leg behind you. Your right arm is forward for counterbalance (Photo 6). **Keep your chest forward and chin down to protect your lower back.** Lightly bounce and swing your left leg behind you, landing on your right. Your left arm comes forward for counterbalance. During workout, emphasis was on contracting the gluteals and lifting the rear leg. But during warm-down, bend the rear leg and emphasize lowering the body deeply over the supporting leg to stretch the gluteal muscles.

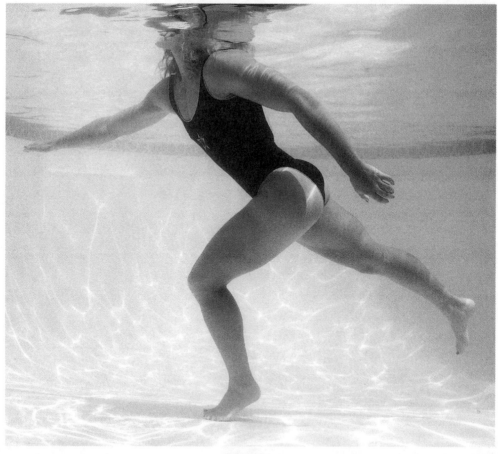

The
Complete
Waterpower
Workout
Book

206

Emphasize bending your front leg, lowering yourself deeply into the water. You can bend your rear leg as well.

Exercise 7. Frog Jumps

Stretch and loosen your hip rotators, gluteals, and adductors with this exercise.

Sit low in the water as you bounce in place on both feet. Then, without jumping, simply lift both knees toward your chest (Photo 7A). *Stay low in the water.* After fifteen repetitions, open the knees wide to the sides and perform another fifteen reps (Photo 7B).

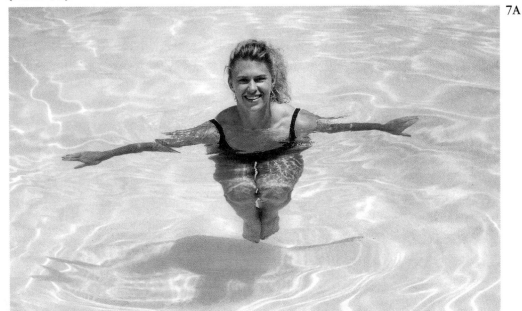

7A

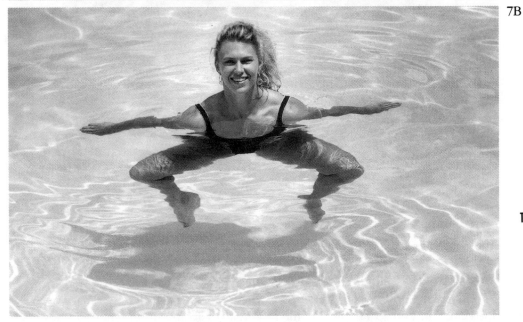

7B

**The Waterpower
Warm-Down**

Exercise 8. Kicking

If you have any residual soreness in your legs, you will feel it and work it out with these kicking variations.

Turn your back to the wall of the pool and brace yourself with your arms on the edge of the pool. If the pool has a step, sit on it as Gea Johnson does in Photo 8. Lift your hips and straight legs and begin gently flutter kicking. Count one repetition for each right/left cycle. Then bend your knees and lightly kick in a bicycling movement. Pull each knee toward your chest easily and rhythmically.

Turn over and face the pool wall. Hold on to the gutter, ladder, step, or side of the pool, and extend your legs behind you. Your face is out of the water. With straight legs, kick fifteen reps.

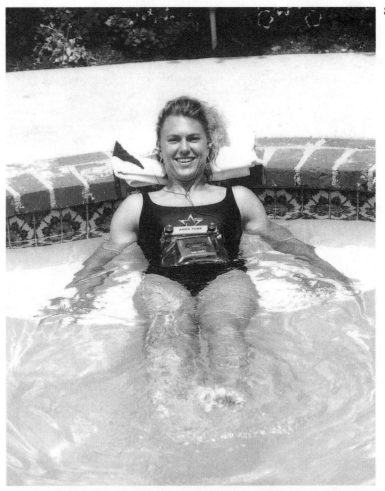

8

The
Complete
Waterpower
Workout
Book

208

You have completed The Waterpower Warm-Down circuit the first time. Now repeat the circuit, this time straightening the legs more, reaching further on each movement.

DEEP WATERPOWER WARM-DOWN

These exercises are virtually the same as their counterparts in The Deep Waterpower Workout, Chapter 3.

Follow the tips below for maximum loosening and stretching:

- Move slowly.
- Emphasize range of motion instead of power.
- Stretch and loosen the body; don't create more work load.
- Begin each movement cautiously and slowly. If you encounter soreness, continue moving at a reduced pace while gradually reaching for full range of motion.

Put on your favorite flotation device (see pages 85 and 86). **Spend two minutes slowly performing each of the exercises listed below.**

Exercise 9. Water Running *(Exercise 1, page 88)*

Exercise 10. Water Walking *(Exercise 2, page 90)*

Exercise 11. Flies *(Exercise 10, page 101)*

Exercise 12. V Kicks *(Exercise 11, page 102)*

Exercise 13. Scissors *(Exercise 22, page 111)*

Exercise 14. Kicking *(See Exercise 8, facing page 208)*

For further recovery after either of the Waterpower Warm-Downs, stretch any sore muscles. Then apply ice to the prime muscles used in your normal activity. Icing causes a shrinking or vasoconstriction of the blood vessels, assisting the return of the blood toward the heart. Ice also reduces edema, the natural collection of fluids in the tissues surrounding the blood vessels that occurs during exercise.

Ideally you should move to the pool and your Waterpower Warm-Down immediately after your run, cycle, or session in the gym. But even if hours go by, or the entire day, your body will still thank you if you can slide into water's magical freshness some time before the day is out.

People often think that heat soothes the muscles after exercise because it feels so good; however, heat causes further vasodilation of the blood vessels, adding to the blood already pooled in the extremities. Furthermore, heat increases swelling and inflammation associated with strenuous workouts. So **choose the cool water of the swimming pool for your water warm-down rather than the heat of the Jacuzzi.** Following the warm-down, you can apply a sophisticated sports medicine technique of contrast baths to promote ultimate recovery: Sit in the Jacuzzi or stand in a hot shower for two minutes; then move to the pool or cold tub for four minutes. Repeat three times, *always* ending with the coolest water to leave the circulatory system in a state of vasoconstriction.

Music motivates nearly everyone, so try putting your sports Walkman into a watertight **Aqua Tunes** case so you can listen to your favorite cassette as you do your Waterpower Warm-Down. (Photo 8, page 208) The Aqua Tunes molded plastic pouch and watertight clamp attach to an adjustable nylon webbed belt to go around your waist. The water-proof earplug speaker system, which comes in two sizes to fit various ears, helps secure the speaker in the ear and seal out water. Although originally designed to break up the boredom for lap swimmers, Aqua Tunes can add another layer of enjoyment for water-training enthusiasts, too. **Carefully read all safety and waterproofing instructions.**

The
Complete
Waterpower
Workout
Book

210

II

Water Healing

S e v e n

Understanding Injury and Healing

I n recent years, the treatment of sports injuries has evolved into a sophisticated science. Injuries that were once disabling are being aggressively rehabilitated, allowing athletes to return quickly and dramatically to competition. In fact, some of these treatments appear to be "miracles."

Water Healing is one of these miracles used in rehabilitating a whole range of sprains, strains, dislocations, and fractures. Following an injury or surgery, Water Healing exercises can begin sooner than traditional physical therapy, thereby cutting down recovery time. And recovery time is vital! Elite athletes often have enormous financial motivation to regain full function, and many recreational athletes feel the drive to speed their healing even though the motivation is strictly emotional. The healing procedures that work for Olympians are equally valuable for recreational athletes and the general fitness-oriented population. Even those who aren't interested in sports, but simply desire a speedy return to their daily life activities, are wisely using water's healing power.

Before turning to a discussion of water's miraculous role in injury rehabilitation, it's helpful to know some of the physiological facts about injury and healing.

Injury and the Inflammatory Response

Injuries fall into two broad categories: macrotrauma and microtrauma. **Macrotrauma** involves abrupt tissue damage either from external impact or internal forces. A torn ligament in the knee from a fall while skiing, a broken leg from a crushing football tackle, a sprained ankle on the tennis court, or a dislocated shoulder while wrestling are all examples of macrotrauma. **Microtrauma** is the repetitive stress placed on tissues over time that results in a cumulative injury. The minor pain at the onset of common overuse injuries such as shin splints, tennis elbow, and tendinitis is an example of microtrauma that left unattended eventually leads to dysfunctional injuries.

Whether an injury is caused by macro- or microtrauma, the result is an inflammatory reaction. The events that follow are similar in all injuries: When tissue is first damaged, the acute inflammatory response causes the smallest surrounding blood vessels, the capillaries, to expand, resulting in an increased volume and pressure of blood within them. Simultaneously, the capillaries become more permeable, that is, the cell walls allow fluid and healing agents to leak more easily into the damaged tissue. These fluids and healing agents are responsible for cleaning up the debris of the injury and reconstructing the injury site. This **acute** inflammatory reaction is usually complete in two weeks. If the reaction continues for one month, it is called a **subacute** inflammation; if it continues for months or years, it has become a **chronic** inflammation.

Although inflammation causes swelling, they are not the same thing. Inflammation is a natural reaction to an injury as described above, but swelling (edema) is a controllable by-product of inflammation. In fact, excessive swelling extends the damage by closing off capillaries neighboring the injury site, thereby starving healthy tissues of nutrients and oxygen.

Swelling should be treated aggressively and early.

The P.R.I.C.E. of an Injury

The livelihood of professional and Olympic athletes depends on injury-free performance. They know that when even the smallest injury occurs, they must pay the **P.R.I.C.E.** immediately.

Protection: Protect against further injury by immobilizing or bracing the injured part during daily activities.

Rest: Immediately cease using the affected area until movement is pain free.

Ice: Surround the injury with an abundance of ice to prevent or diminish the expansion of the capillaries that leads to swelling. Apply ice for ten to twenty minutes every waking hour during the first forty-eight hours, then twice a day until the injury is resolved.

Compression: Immediately apply pressure to the involved area with tape, an Ace bandage, or an air-compression sleeve. Compression helps prevent swelling or the leakage of excess fluids into the tissues.

The
Complete
Waterpower
Workout
Book

214

Elevation: Keep the injury raised higher than the heart, promoting the drainage of whatever fluids do leak into the tissues surrounding the injury. In this way, swelling is kept to a minimum.

P.R.I.C.E. dictates the actions of professional and Olympic athletes in the first crucial phase of an injury as it should yours.

Healing

The inflammatory response continues, and approximately one week after the injury a healing repair stage begins. It is characterized by an increase in the number of cells that lay down scar tissue known as granulation. At approximately the end of the second week, the remodeling phase begins in which the maturation of this scar tissue occurs. At this point, gentle appropriate movement can help build a strong, functional scar less likely to be reinjured. But while gentle, active exercises focused on improving range of motion can stimulate the proper remodeling of the scar tissue, **excessive force in exercise will disrupt healing or cause reinjury.** Water is the ideal medium in which to perform these early range-of-motion exercises.

Most injuries are considered stable after six weeks. The completion of the healing process may take many months or even a full year and is characterized by the return to normal function and formation of a mature scar. Yet the area surrounding the injury has become deconditioned. The goal of all rehabilitation is to eliminate dysfunction and return the body to a preinjury (or better) state of fitness. Once initial healing has been achieved by adherence to the P.R.I.C.E. principles the rehabilitative process is ready to begin with early safe exercise.

Water: The New Therapy

Until recently, conventional wisdom dictated that injured areas of the body should be immobilized for long periods. Now, however, exercise is considered a healing agent by most doctors and physical therapists, because therapists create in a clinical setting what the body does as a matter of course during exercise. Heat packs cause vasodilation; so does exercise. Acupuncture and TENS units stimulate the release of endorphins to fight pain, and so does exercise. Ultrasound and micro-electrical current devices increase cellular metabolism and activate healing mechanisms. So does exercise. Finally, ice reduces pain and diminishes muscle spasms, and so does exercise.

Thus exercise can help speed healing, and the best place to exercise is in the water. Many progressive rehabilitation programs today include early movement in water to prevent or minimize the secondary-damage events that occur after an injury, such as stiffening, loss of circulation, an involvement of other body parts surrounding the injury, and muscle atrophy (loss of muscle size). In this way, early-movement water programs promote quicker resolution of an injury. As the healing process continues, early-

Ice: Frozen Waterpower

Ice is life's most underrecognized drug and it needs no prescription. It's right there waiting for you in your freezer. It's quick and easy to apply to an injury, quick to start working.

When an injury occurs, immediate application of ice constricts the capillaries, to help prevent bleeding and swelling in the injured area and creating a bruise. The use of ice decreases the need for antipain medication. Ice serves as a counterirritant, a surface stimulus that overrides the pain in the injured area. It acts as a painkiller also by raising the threshold of the nerves that signal when you're in pain. Ice slows nerve conduction velocity. In plain words, ice shuts down many nerve impulses that your brain interprets as pain.

Apply lavish amounts of ice to your injury and the area surrounding it. Use a large ice bag. Or fill a towel with ice cubes and fold it to create a bag. Using a wet towel or ice bag keeps the ice from directly touching your skin, which can cause burns.

Leave the ice bag in place ten to twenty minutes, then remove it and wrap a dry towel around the cold skin until you feel the area thaw. Wait ten minutes and ice your injury again. Ice on and off as often as possible during the first two days of your injury, then reduce this treatment to twice a day until the injury heals.

In treating neck and back injuries, ice is applied to alleviate pain, spasm, or inflammation even though the initial discomfort of the cold may give the impression of stiffening the muscles. As long as you stay relaxed as you ice, the muscles will not shorten; ice treatment actually allows muscles that are in spasm to relax and return to their normal resting length.

For convenience, complete mobility, and adjustable compression, **ICE 'N' HEAT** can be used instead of ice bags. ICE 'N' HEAT consists of a freezable gel pack, insulated soft fabric wrap, and an elastic extension belt. The elastic belt holds the

movement programs have been proven to stimulate the rapid formation of stronger, more functional scar tissue.

Traditionally, therapists utilize primarily nonweight-bearing exercises to isolate and strengthen injured links in the body chain. For instance, to strengthen a knee following surgery, patients do quad extensions and hamstring curls, which isolate the function of these muscles at the knee joint. These exercises are examples of an **"open kinetic chain,"** meaning that during them, movement systems are open at one end. In this case, although the leg pushes against the resistance of weights, the foot moves freely in space; it does not operate under the weight of the body. Water is an ideal medium for open kinetic chain exercises. The Deep Waterpower Workout provides such exercises during suspended work. These open kinetic chain exercises are a means of strengthening the

The
Complete
Waterpower
Workout
Book

216

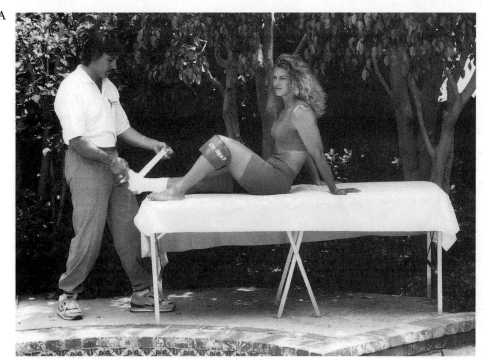

A

Robert Forster, P.T., ices Gea Johnson's knee and tapes her ankle to protect it during a Waterpower Workout.

gel pack in the most desirable position over your arm or leg injury (see Photo A), or extends so you can use it around your lower back or shoulders. You can wrap the ICE 'N' HEAT ice bag snugly around any injury and continue your daily activities at home or work. (Once you've passed the first forty-eight hours of your injury, ICE 'N' HEAT's gel pack can go into the microwave and be heated to offer contrast treatments—first cold, then heat, then *always* finish with cold.)

weakest link in the body system before attempting to have several parts of the body function together as they will upon their return to full activity. Of course, in the real world of sport, joints never work in isolation. Instead, the joints operate together and augment each other's function. For example, in running, as the foot contacts the ground in the running stride, the joints of the foot, ankle, knee, and hip function sequentially under the load of the body weight to provide efficient human movement. This is an example of a **"closed kinetic chain"** movement (a weight-bearing movement) in which the force created at each heel strike closes that end of the chain. The Waterpower Workout in Chapter 2 contains closed kinetic chain exercises.

The newest direction in rehabilitation of lower-limb sports injuries involves *early* performance of closed kinetic chain (weight-bearing) exercises to closely simulate actual land-based sports activities. A possible drawback with this new approach is the introduction of weight-bearing exercises before the injured link in the system is strong enough to handle the load of body weight, which can disrupt healing or create further injury. Therefore, the addition of closed kinetic exercises is a critical point in the rehab process and should not begin until such movement is pain free. In water, these potentially dangerous movements become safer because water's buoyancy makes the body 90 percent weightless in shoulder-deep water. This means closed kinetic chain exercises can safely be introduced much earlier in water than on land. As the body recovers and the rehabilitation progresses, weight bearing in closed kinetic chain exercises increases by moving to shallower water. Flotation devices can be worn in shallow water to provide further modulation and control of weight-bearing forces. **Before proceeding, see your doctor for an accurate diagnosis of your injury.**

Water Healing Workout

The Water Healing Workout, by design, doesn't focus solely on your injury and its rehabilitation. Rather, it pulls together the **specific rehabilitation exercises** you must perform to regain full function of your injured area and combines them with a progressive, protective **fitness program.** This combined rehab plus fitness workout perfectly satisfies the first tenet of sports medicine: **Preserve as much fitness and function as possible while rehabilitating an injury.** During Water Healing, you may actually *improve* your fitness level. As your entire body becomes stronger, it moves with greater ease. As you reduce excess weight you may have carried, your injury isn't so severely stressed with every step. Thus improved fitness speeds your overall recovery.

Water Healing Workouts satisfy all the goals of a complete sports rehabilitation program. They turn what seems like a negative experience—an injury—into a positive result: improved strength, increased flexibility, better biomechanics, more endurance, and greater balance. The later stages of rehab that are normally dedicated to redeveloping overall fitness are shortened because you've been maintaining your fitness throughout your rehab. In fact, all the stages may be shortened as your rehab goals are achieved more rapidly in water. The end result is that you are back to your sport and daily activities more quickly.

Water Healing Workouts are particularly indicated for anyone suffering from an injury where there is:

- decreased range of motion or strength;
- pain during movement against gravity;
- lack of coordination on land;
- difficulty when walking or running;
- lack of aerobic or anaerobic capacity;
- a need for early movement in a gravity-neutral environment.

Before beginning a water healing program you should consult with your doctor or physical therapist. As with all therapy, certain precautions must be taken

The
Complete
Waterpower
Workout
Book

218

for safety reasons or to prevent an increase in symptoms. Here are the few circumstances in which Water Healing Workouts should *not* be attempted:

- open wounds or sores;
- a cast that is not waterproof;
- contagious skin conditions;
- allergies to pool chemicals;
- fever;
- urinary tract infections;
- sutures not yet removed (unless surgeon approves);
- uncontrolled seizures;
- doctor or therapist disapproval.

Wait until any of these conditions have ceased before first entering the water.

If an injury brought you to these pages, read through the entire book before beginning your Water Healing Workout. You'll need to have a basic understanding of the exercises in chapters 2 and 3 in order to put together your own session in chapters 8 through 10. If you are recovering from surgery, also see Chapter 11 for special Postsurgical Water Healing.

The Emotional Aspects of Injury

While injury and healing are physical processes, they are usually accompanied by many strong emotions. Whether you are in training for the Olympics or you are a weekend athlete, being sidelined by injury can be a very upsetting experience. Here are some suggestions to see you through it.

Don't panic. Panic causes you to make bad decisions, increases your sense of gloom, and according to holistic doctors, can actually slow down the healing process. When you stay calm, you think more clearly, you retain your emotional balance, and you ensure better decision making. When you know you have a viable exercise alternative, it's easier to stay calm. Simply switch to your water gear, and continue your workouts, keeping in mind the P.R.I.C.E. principles outlined earlier.

You don't have to stop working out. Injuries to the lower body can dramatically change your daily life. Immediately following traumatic injuries, you may not be able to walk from one room to another. Every step becomes a major maneuver. Yet in deep water, you can run, walk, and actively exercise. You can leave your crutches or wheelchair poolside, and for at least an hour a day you won't feel disabled. (Even people in casts can enter the pool these days. Ask your doctor for a removable cast, or a fiberglass cast with a waterproof lining.)

First, you must protect the injured area. With your injury immobilized, you can continue to train the rest of your body. Read chapters 8, 9, 10, and 11, before beginning a Water Healing Workout.

Use your convalescent time wisely. Now is the time to strengthen any weak areas in your fitness program. Look over the nine aspects of fitness on pages 11 through 13. Work on your weaknesses while you train in the water to maintain your present fitness level. Besides your body, there may be weak spots in your life. Consider ways to better balance your physical, mental, financial, emotional, and spiritual worlds.

Learn about your injury. Find out what has been injured and why. Learning what has happened to your muscles, tendons, ligaments, bones, or joints will help you understand the reason for doing each exercise. Then, as you begin your Water Healing Workout, you will be able accurately to visualize the muscles and connective tissue becoming stronger, the bones knitting, the joints becoming sturdy again.

Decide whether you must alter your training program to avoid future similar injuries. Consider whether yours is an overtraining injury. Did you receive warning signals such as insomnia, loss of appetite, nervousness? If so, learn your lesson so you can identify the overtraining circumstance *before* injury strikes again.

Establish a routine and stick with it. Go through the process set forth in Chapter 8 of building your Water Healing Workout. If you need more guidance, find a water exercise coach or therapist to help you devise your personal plan and supervise your first few sessions. Then schedule a time that fits comfortably into your daily life with the least possible conflict. Even on days when you want to stay home and brood, make the effort to go to the pool. Consistency is the prime ingredient in progressing rapidly toward full function again. Once you know your routine, find a training partner to meet you for workouts. You'll be less likely to miss or be late to a session if you know someone is waiting for you.

Reevaluate your eating habits. While training hard, you may have gotten away with some borderline eating practices. Perhaps you craved salt, so you ate a bag of potato chips every afternoon. Or maybe you devoured an entire box of chocolate mints in the movies. (A top marathoner once said, "If the fire is hot enough, it will burn anything.") Now is the time to carefully scrutinize those habits and pull in the reins. During rehabilitation, you will probably be burning fewer calories, so you need to think of "prescribing" nutritious food to yourself that will accelerate your healing process. Eliminate all recreational foods.

Feel and sense the work *you can do* as you mindfully monitor your body. Healing is what the body is programmed for; healing is what the body does best. Savor each physical accomplishment in your Water Healing Workout, no matter how small it seems. By focusing on what is positive, you maintain a better attitude and give your body its best chance for bouncing back quickly. Don't even think about what you can't do.

If you experience extreme frustration, anger, or depression, try adding yoga or meditation to your routine. Many recreational athletes are exercise junkies. They need their emotional "fix" from endurance training. If this describes you, and even the most powerful water exercise session doesn't quench the need for *your* activity, the need isn't purely physical. Use this time for introspection and getting to know the deeper sides of yourself. Yoga and meditation are excellent ways to find calmness and inner growth during difficult times.

The
Complete
Waterpower
Workout
Book

220

E i g h t

Designing
Your Water Healing
Workout

The Water Healing Workout you will design for yourself in this chapter will be composed of exercises from the workouts described in chapters 2 and 3 and specific rehabilitation exercises for the area you have injured. Successful rehabilitation depends on performing exercises that are appropriate to your stage of recovery. Doing exercises before your body is ready for them can cause reinjury and slow the healing process. Before designing your workout, first consult your doctor or physical therapist, then familiarize yourself with the four phases of rehabilitation described below. Learn what precautions to take, and goals to strive for in each. If you do, you will enjoy the full power of water's healing magic.

The Four Phases of Rehabilitation

PHASE 1

Immediately after an injury, you will find yourself in the first phase of rehabilitation. This phase will last one to three weeks and is characterized by the following:

1. **Pain.** Moderate to severe pain is nearly constant on a daily basis. Pain can be present while engaging in daily activities or only during sports participation. All pain is caused by inflammation.

2. **Inflammation.** Injured tissues release chemical irritants that stimulate nerve impulses relaying pain or creating the pain experience. Inflammation causes swelling.

3. **Swelling (Edema).** Swelling occurs as the body attempts to reach a state of equilibrium between the fluid in the blood vessels and the fluid within the tissues of an injury site. As healing agents gather around the injury, fluid leaves the blood vessels to dilute what has become highly concentrated fluid in the injured tissues. Hence, swelling. Swelling causes more pain as it puts pressure on the nerves. It closes down capillaries, prevents adequate circulation to the uninjured tissues around the injury, and therefore causes additional tissue to die from lack of oxygen (apoxia). Swelling causes a loss of mobility.

4. **Loss of mobility.** Pressure within a joint or tissue caused by swelling makes moving that area difficult. Further, pain stimulates "splinting," increased muscular contraction in the area to protect a joint.

5. **Loss of function.** When mobility is lost in muscles, joints, and connective tissues, they also lose function. Muscles will be inhibited (less likely to contract) due to the pain and swelling and start to atrophy (shrink) literally within hours. In fact, each day of immobility produces a 1.5 percent loss in muscle size and stamina. The first muscle fibers to begin to deteriorate are the "fast-twitch" fibers responsible for speed and power. Joint stiffness quickly develops when muscles surrounding joints are in the protective "splinting" mode. When connective tissue is inflamed, it develops adhesions that can lead to a more permanent loss of mobility.

6. **Rapid deterioration of fitness level.** Without function or mobility, you lose fitness. Unless some activity is maintained, hard-earned fitness gains quickly decline.

The goals of Phase 1 are to begin to resolve all of the above occurrences; however, the major emphasis is on improving mobility while eliminating pain, inflammation, and swelling. All six factors can be addressed in the water. Pain is reduced, because the stimulation of the water overrides pain to some degree. Once in the water, you can begin movement. Movement creates competing nerve impulses that also override pain. The cooling effect of water causes vasoconstriction (constriction of the blood vessels) and through a complex series of events eliminates the chemical products of inflammation. Swelling is reduced by gentle movement, by the water's coolness and by the hydrostatic pressure (the pressure the water exerts evenly over the entire surface of the submerged body). In water you will quickly regain your lost mobility. You will be able to perform

The
Complete
Waterpower
Workout
Book

222

motions in the water *much sooner* than you could on land. When your recovery activities are carried out in the water, you prevent possible aggravation or reinjury and therefore further loss of function. By protecting the injured area and performing Water Healing Workouts, you will be able to achieve the goals of Phase 1 while you retain your fitness level. **Tape, brace, or cast your injury and get in the pool as soon as your doctor or physical therapist will allow.** Do whatever gentle exercises you can tolerate. And because this may be the only movement you can currently do, do it daily. If you perform your Water Healing Workouts daily or every two days, you will usually be ready to move to Phase 2 in seven to ten days. Whether you exercise daily or not, ice twice a day. Whether you think icing is helping or not, **keep icing.** (See page 216 for details on icing).

Until pain, inflammation, and swelling are checked, you cannot move on to Phase 2.

PHASE 2

You enter Phase 2 when you can identify your first significant reduction of symptoms and improvement in function: less pain, increased range of motion, and the ability to contract your muscles fully. Phase 2 usually lasts three to six weeks and is characterized by minimal to moderate intermittent pain that comes from movement such as the activities of daily living, certain postures, or sports activity. Moderate inflammation and swelling are still present, and a moderate loss of mobility and function still exist, but **symptoms have begun to decrease.** It is time to begin regaining strength and establishing the base for more strenuous rehabilitation to follow.

The goals of Phase 2 continue to be the reduction of whatever pain, inflammation, and swelling remain, but the major thrust of this phase is to continue improving flexibility and begin increasing strength. Because you are able to move around more in daily life and can work harder in each Water Healing Workout, you can either continue daily sessions, or you can cut back to a minimum of four sessions a week. In the following pages you will learn of the various components that will make up your Water Healing Workout. Continue to wear protective taping or bracing during the fitness portion, and increase the intensity of your intervals. You may now remove such protection during your specific rehabilitation exercises you will select from chapters 9, 10, and 11 if you can do the exercises without pain. If pain caused you to begin in deep water (open kinetic chain), try to move to the shallow-water (closed kinetic chain) exercises during this phase. Add a flotation device to increase your buoyancy as needed to prevent pain upon impact.

PHASE 3

Phase 3 lasts anywhere from one to three months, depending on the injury. By this time you should be experiencing only minimal intermittent pain that occurs solely during activity. All other symptoms should be minimal as well. The emphasis during Phase 3 is to regain full strength, flexibility, aerobic and anaerobic fitness, and the skills necessary to return to sports training, but not competition.

It is during this phase that many people commonly become stuck, not reaching their goals on the road to the recovery. Too often people don't appreciate the subtle goals that must be achieved during Phase 3, and they abandon their rehab program for a premature full return to land. The almost imperceptible swelling, chronic inflammation, incomplete range of motion, and decrease in strength are the last traces of the injury, but they are very real obstacles to regaining full function. If these problems are not resolved, an early return to full sports participation often results in entering a frustrating cycle of injury and reinjury.

During this phase, resolve the cause of the injury as well. Focus on changing the training patterns or biomechanics that may have contributed to your injury. Since you have resumed *some, but not all,* of your land training, continue doing three Water Healing Workouts a week.

PHASE 4

Phase 4 means that you no longer have any symptoms. You are ready to return to full training in order to return to competition. The rule of thumb is that you should be pain free in your sports training and should have recovered 95 percent of your strength and flexibility before resuming competition or performance. You may take between two and four weeks in Phase 4 to reach that level. When you return to competition, retain one water day a week in your training program for several months or indefinitely. Perform The Waterpower Workout program (Chapter 2) and work your way up to Level 3 or The Twenty-five-Minute Powerhouse Workout. Congratulate yourself: You are no longer doing Water Healing; you are all the way back to Waterpower.

How to Build Your
Water Healing Workout

When you are injured, some of the exercises you learned in The Waterpower and Deep Waterpower Workouts may cause you pain. Virtually all of the shallow-water exercises would aggravate a weight-bearing injury, so if you have a foot, leg, hip, or back injury eliminate Chapter 2 at first. But even some of the Deep Waterpower Workout exercises in Chapter 3 may cause you pain. Your job is to slowly and carefully try each one and determine which exercises would aggravate your injury and which exercises you can do without pain. Make the **painless** exercises part of your program. Use this guide: If pain does not decrease as you perform the repititions of your first set of an exercise, you are disrupting the healing and possibly aggravating the injury.

Once you have compiled your list of painless Waterpower and Deep Waterpower exercises, you will add the other components of a Water Healing Workout listed below. Plan on spending at least thirty minutes maintaining your fitness, then additional time addressing the rehabilitation of your injury.

Your thirty-five- to sixty-minute Water Healing Workout will be assembled from the following components. After reading this chapter and chapters 9, 10, and 11, you will

The
Complete
Waterpower
Workout
Book

224

choose the ones appropriate to your injury and fitness level. You will choose *only one* of fitness components 4, 5, 6, or 7 as you begin Water Healing, but as you progress, you may have exercises from several in your program.

1. Deep-Water Running and Walking Warm-Up	5 minutes
2. Stretching	3 to 5 minutes
3. Deep-Water Intervals	0 to 10 minutes
4. The Deep Waterpower Workout or	0 to 10 minutes
5. The Waterpower Warm-Down or	0 to 15 minutes
6. The Waterpower Workout or	0 to 45 minutes
7. The Twenty-five-Minute Powerhouse Workout	0 to 25 minutes
8. Gait Training	0 to 10 minutes
9. Specific Rehabilitation Exercises (SREs)	5 to 15 minutes
10. Resistance Training	0 to 10 minutes
11. Sport-Specific or Dance-Specific Waterpower Workouts	0 to 20 minutes

(Those who love to swim can replace components 1 and 3 with ten to twenty minutes of crawl, backstroke, or the assisted swimming exercises on pages 256 through 260.

Dancers recovering from an injury should read all the guidelines and cautions in this chapter before turning back to Dance-Specific Waterpower Workouts in Chapter 4.) Descriptions of each of these components are provided below.

1. **Deep-Water Running and Walking Warm-Up.** (Exercises 1 and 2, pages 88 to 90.) If you have knee pain, you may have to eliminate the running, or perform it very slowly. If you have lower back pain, the walking may hurt. But **virtually everyone can do one or the other.** Begin slowly, monitoring how your injury feels and how the rest of your body feels. Start with a three-minute warm-up run or a two-minute warm-up walk. (Remember that water walking is harder than water running.) If you can both water run and water walk without pain, do both. Even when you progress to shallow water for the bulk of your exercises, do your warm-up in deep water.

2. **Stretch.** Turn back to the side of the pool and grasp a ladder, gutter, railing, or skimmer box. If your pool has none of these features, and if holding the lip of the pool is uncomfortable, consider buying two Hol-Tite restrainers (Photo 27, page 116) to make your stretching easier. Attempt each of the following stretches carefully and slowly. If you experience pain, decrease the stretch to eliminate the pain and hold the new position while you relax and breathe deeply. You may not be able to do every exercise below without pain. Skip any exercise that causes pain and attempt it even more gently in the next Water Healing Workout.
Curl and Stretch (Exercise 27, page 116)
Body Swing (Exercise 28, page 117)
Hamstring Stretch (Exercise 26, page 115)

Quad Stretch (Exercise 25, page 114)
Triangle (Exercise 30, page 66)

3. **Deep-Water Intervals.** Follow the Level 1, 2, or 3 interval training programs set forth in Chapter 3, exercises 3 and 8.

4. **The Deep Waterpower Workout.** Do these suspended exercises if yours is a weight-bearing injury. As you progress through your rehab phases (see charts in chapters 9, 10, and 11), you will move to shallow-water programs. If your rehab phase dictates that you use Deep Waterpower, *gently* try Exercise 4, page 94. (You have already warmed up with Exercises 1 and 2, and may have already performed the Deep-Water Intervals of Exercise 3. If you can perform Exercise 4 with no pain, put it in your Water Healing Workout. If you must seriously modify the exercise in order to do it without pain, it shouldn't be part of your program. Move on to each exercise in the entire Deep Waterpower series. Those exercises that cause you pain or discomfort should be skipped for now. Select only those exercises you feel comfortable doing and eliminate those you question. (Lists of exercises that are normally avoided because of specific injuries or postsurgical conditions appear throughout Chapters 9, 10, and 11. If you try those exercises, be especially slow and careful.)

    Create a list of the exercises that will make up your current program. Stick with these same exercises for the first week of Water Healing, then go through the selection process again, adding any new exercises that no longer cause discomfort or pain. (See box on page 232 as an example of the exercises selected by a UCLA athlete with a knee injury.) Every week, try again until you're able to perform all or nearly all of the Deep Waterpower exercises. As you move through the phases of your rehabilitation, the charts in Chapters 9, 10, and 11 direct you to move on to shallow-water programs.

5. **The Waterpower Warm-Down.** As soon as you can tolerate gentle weight bearing, you will move to the shallow-water Waterpower Warm-Down program (Chapter 6), in which all exercises are designed to be slow and gentle. You can increase your buoyancy, thereby reducing impact, by wearing a flotation device in shallow water. *Gently* try Exercise 1, then 2, and so on until you select all those you can do without pain. Put those in your current program, replacing several of your easiest Deep Waterpower exercises.

6. **The Waterpower Workout.** As your ability to tolerate weight bearing (and bouncing) increases, you will progress to the more strenuous Waterpower Workout, Chapter 2. Again, try each exercise, and add all pain-free exercises to your current Water Healing Workout. Eliminate each Waterpower Warm-Down exercise as soon as you can painlessly do the similar Waterpower Workout version. As you add more and more shallow-water exercises, you will begin phasing out the Deep Waterpower exercises, keeping only the warm-up at the deep end of the pool. This gradual transition to shallow water best prepares you for the return to land.

7. **The Twenty-five-Minute Powerhouse Workout.** Just before your return to land, you will want to test your body's ability to jump high and work hard with this high-intensity program. See page 78.

The
Complete
Waterpower
Workout
Book

226

8. **Gait Training.** If your weight-bearing injury has put you on crutches or altered your gait pattern, you can relearn correct walking biomechanics in chest-deep water. A limp caused by an injury can become a habit. You must teach yourself to walk again with balance and strength. See exercises 24 through 27 in Chapter 9, pages 264 to 267.

9. **Specific Rehabilitation Exercises (SREs).** When you first begin your Water Healing Workout, you may have to skip this segment. Your injury may be too acutely inflamed and therefore should be totally immobilized. On the other hand, you may be able to begin immediately. Slowly test each of the SREs and perform only those you can do with minimal or no pain. If you cannot do any of the SREs, begin by protecting your injury and continuing to train the rest of your body while the injury begins the first stages of its healing processes. Then, over the following weeks, you will begin introducing specific exercises designed to bring back full range of motion and strength to your injury site. This work will increase as you progress through the four phases of rehabilitation and your sets and reps build. The SREs can be found in chapters 9 and 10. Find your injured body part and read the exercises to be incorporated into your workout. If you are building a Postsurgical Water Healing Workout, your SREs are in Chapter 11.

A

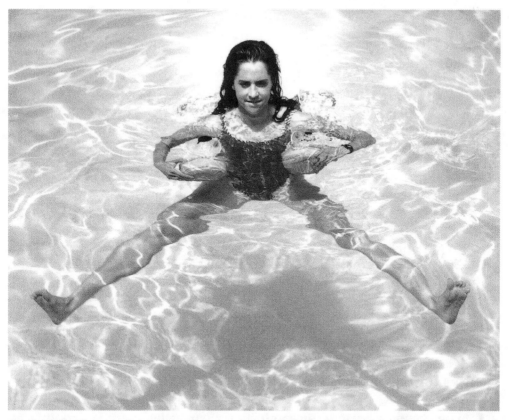

One SpaBell with Dome Cap under each arm provides stability for the shoulders while you do lower body exercises.

Various pieces of equipment will give you exactly the body position or the buoyancy that you'll need. See the list of equipment at the end of this chapter and in the Appendix.

10. **Resistance Training.** While your injury is healing, you can use resistance equipment to strengthen the *other* parts of your body. Then, during Phase 3 of your rehab, you will add resistance equipment as you perform your SREs. Adding extra resistance is similar to increasing the weight you lift in the weight room to induce strength gains. You can gradually move from slight resistance to forceful resistance equipment. (See equipment descriptions at the end of this chapter and listings of where to find them in the Appendix.) As you use this equipment, you will automatically be slowed in your movements. This gives you more time for increased muscle involvement for every repetition. Don't push for speed yet. Muscle, tendon, or other soft-tissue strains are possible if these pieces are used prematurely or with too much force.

11. **Sport-Specific or Dance-Specific Waterpower Workouts.** Once you have completed the bulk of your Water Healing Workout, including the rehab work specific to your injury, then work at maintaining the timing and skill in your sport or dance. Choose the exercises that precisely emulate your land-based activity as detailed in Chapters 4 and 5.

Tips for Water Therapy

When doing your Water Healing Workout, keep these guidelines in mind:

- **Protect the injured area.** This may mean taping a sprained ankle or putting a waterproof brace on your knee. With the injured area immobilized, you can work the uninjured body parts to retain or to build fitness. At the first stages of your water rehab program, you will concentrate on total body fitness while ignoring (and immobilizing) the injury. Once you can tolerate movement in the injured area, you will spend more time doing specific rehabilitation exercises.

- **Differentiate between the fitness and specific rehab portions of your Water Healing Workout.** Eliminate all exercises that cause pain during the **fitness portion** of your session. But you will probably experience some pain as you do the **specific rehab exercises.** This pain is unavoidable as you learn the edges of your ever-changing limitations. Each session you will reach to the edge, feel some pain, and pull back to a safe range of motion. When you know where the "red line" is for pain-free movement on a particular day, do not cross that red line. If you do this conscientiously, you won't aggravate the injury and you will be able to do the specific rehab work to increase your mobility and strength in the injured joint or tissues.

- **If you encounter pain or discomfort on a particular exercise, modify it by moving more slowly. If that doesn't eliminate the pain, narrow the range of motion.** Your body's pain messages are the best guide you have for setting up your Water Healing Workout. Listen carefully. When working alone, without the

The
Complete
Waterpower
Workout
Book

228

help of a doctor, coach, or therapist, keep this guideline in mind: **If it hurts, don't do it.**

- **If you can't yet move the injured joint, begin by moving the adjacent joints.** Many muscles cross two joints and therefore cause movement at both joints. For example, the gastrocnemius (calf) muscle crosses both the ankle and the knee. If your ankle is damaged and you can't flex and extend it, keep strength in the gastroc by working it from the other end, at the knee, by performing exercises that flex the knee. Other examples of muscles that cross two joints are the quadriceps and hamstrings (hip and knee) and the triceps and biceps (shoulder and elbow). By working adjacent body parts in this manner, you can maintain some degree of strength in the damaged area.

- **During the specific rehab exercises, pain and swelling may severely limit the movement at first.** Each time you do your water rehab work, you will feel a little less pain and a little greater mobility.

- **During the fitness portion of your Water Healing session, train as strenuously as you can without causing jarring or discomfort at the injury site.** If you feel pain to the injury, you may have to slow your interval training and other exercises or increase the protection (tape or brace) of the injured area.

- **Perform all Water Healing exercises gently, smoothly, and with correct biomechanics (form).** This may mean asking a therapist, coach, or knowledgeable friend to supervise you until you are sure all movements are exact. Use this time while you are slowed by injury to improve any faulty movement patterns that may have contributed to your injury. General rules of correct biomechanics appear on page 76.

- **Underdo anything new.** Any time you attempt a new movement, begin slowly, monitoring for possible pain. Since you may not feel the pain of a new movement until the next day, perform fewer reps at a slower speed than you think you can tolerate.

- **If you are in the acute phase (Phase 1) of an injury for which surgery was recommended, but you've chosen nonsurgical therapy, see the specific guidelines under your diagnosis in Chapter 11, Postsurgical Water Healing.** Even though you did not have surgery, you should be aware of the precautions that accompany your injury. These precautions will usually be the same whether you have an acute nonsurgical injury or whether you are in the Postsurgical Phase 1.

- **Increase your work load very gradually.** After you've built up to the number of reps recommended in the programs to follow, begin increasing speed, which increases water resistance.

  Toss out the work ethic you may have developed in your sports training. If you feel fatigue setting in and can't decide how much work to complete, remind yourself that you are water healing, not water training. **When in doubt, don't.**

- **Schedule your land therapy and water therapy on alternating days.** If you already have a land-based physical therapy program in place, perform your Water Healing Workout on alternate days so you don't bring undue fatigue with you into the pool. Check with your therapist regarding any Water Healing exercises that you question.

- **Continue to perform your warm-up in deep water to avoid all impact.** Even though you may have progressed so that the majority of your water rehab work is in shallow water, start deep.

- **After a warm-up, stretch the injury site.** As your rehabilitation progresses and your injury can tolerate more movement, you will need to spend more and more time stretching the area to regain full flexibility.

- **Do it first in the water.** If you're a basketball player recovering from an injury and you're not sure if you can tolerate jumping on the court, perform repeated jumps first in the water. If you're an injured dancer wanting to get back on pointe but don't know if your foot can hold your entire body weight, try it first in the water. Whatever new move you wish to make, do it first in the water. If you make a misstep, you can't fall in water. If you really weren't ready yet to try this new move, you won't have as severe a price to pay if you find it out in water.

- **If you have arthritis, multiple sclerosis, muscular dystrophy, or have had a stroke or heart attack, seek medical guidance in setting up your Water Healing Workout.** The programs and exercises in this book focus specifically on musculoskeletal problems, but you will find ideas here that can help your condition as well. Retraining yourself to walk in the water is particularly beneficial. (See Gait Training Exercises 24 to 27, pages 264 through 267.) Other aspects of your program will require additional expertise from your doctor.

- **Find a cold pool to speed healing.** Some health clubs have a small pool filled with cold water (50 to 60 degrees). These are ideal for performing gentle range-of-motion exercises for your injury, especially when pain is dominant in Phase 1. You can make circles with your ankle or wrist, bend and straighten your knee, or bend and arch a sore back. Most cold pools are adjacent to the hot Jacuzzi, so you can perform contrast-bath treatments—cold, hot, cold, hot, *always* ending with cold.

Equipment List

Though water itself is the most important "equipment" you need to maintain your fitness level and rehabilitate your injury, specialized equipment can help you fine-tune your Water Healing Workout by offering you precise body position, buoyancy, or added resistance. See also pages 85 and 86 for flotation equipment.

Aquarius water workout station. This stainless steel multistation unit offers you a seat and various handles and leg-bracing bars for pull-ups, sit-ups, leg lifts, side swings, and a variety of other exercises. (Photos 12 and 13, pages 172 and 173.) Talk to the pool manager about purchasing an Aquarius. Installing one turns a part of your aquatic facility into an effective workout or rehabilitation site. The unit weighs under fifty pounds and can be easily removed for storage. Add-on attachments are available that further enhance its capability.

Aquatoner. The Aquatoner is a versatile resistance tool. Its centrally placed handle is connected with stainless steel hardware through three plastic, spreadable paddles. Opposite the handle is a sturdy Velcro cushion that can be attached to a foot, an ankle,

The
Complete
Waterpower
Workout
Book

230

or an arm. The Aquatoner takes refined neuromuscular coordination to control, which makes it ideal for dancers and athletes who must learn precise technical skill. (See Photo 15D, page 138.)

Bodyciser. This therapeutic, buoyant exercise platform allows you to perform strengthening and stretching movements beneath the water while in a horizontal, vertical, or seated position. The Bodyciser permits unlimited variations and degrees of flexion, extension, and lateral movements, while the head and ears remain out of the water at all times. Exercising on the Bodyciser keeps pressure off your tailbone, vertebrae, and disks, and places your back in a neutral position best for avoiding reaggravation of back problems while strengthening the lower back, abdominal, buttocks, and thigh muscles. Flotation cushions can be added or subtracted to increase or decrease buoyancy and to increase or decrease exercise intensity. This folding aquatic platform weighs six pounds and comes with a strap for easy carrying to the pool. (See photos 35A, 35B, and 38, pages 325 and 327.)

Hydro-Tone. Hydro-Tone bells and boots (see photos C, D, E, and F, pages 193 and 194) most closely approach weight training. Because they interact with the water along all planes, they deliver smooth, stable resistance for all arm and leg movements. These bright yellow plastic pieces never jerk, turn, or wobble as other pieces can that are not three dimensional. The bells are easy to grasp and control through a full range of upper-body exercises. The boots are virtually the only multidimensional resistance piece of equipment for the lower body currently available. Hydro-Tone offers the most vigorous resistance workout of all the equipment.

Instructional Swim Bar. This thirty-inch bar can be used therapeutically for both the upper body and lower body. You can stand on it, creating the lightest version of a closed-kinetic chain for rehabilitating knees, hips, and ankles (See photos 19A and 19B, page 319). You can sit on it to perform noncontact leg exercises. And you can use it against water's buoyancy to create resistance for specific arm, chest, and shoulder rehab work (Photo 5, page 277). The bar can be used to assist nonswimmers in learning to swim.

SpaBells. Dome caps can be snapped onto the funnel ends of SpaBells, trapping air inside so they become flotation devices. A SpaBell with dome caps can be held in each hand or tucked under each arm to stabilize arms or shoulders while you work only the lower body in water walking, water running, or flies (Photo A, page 227). When you remove the dome caps, SpaBells become resistance equipment to be used underwater. They provide three-dimensional, variable resistance to water and they have three different areas of resistance—the funnels, the large vanes, and the small vanes. Resistance can be substantially increased on the SpaBells by adding power vanes (Photo B, page 234). When you use SpaBells, be certain to hold each device exactly the same in each hand for a consistent, balanced feel and to maintain proper control throughout the exercise.

Speedo SwimMitt XT aquatic cross-training gloves. The SwimMitt XT is the first water-training equipment to provide additional resistance both below *and* above the water. The neoprene webbing provides more surface area for pulling through water, yet is more gentle on your shoulders and transfers less stress to your rotator cuff muscles than plastic hand paddles. The open-finger design lets you take your pulse during workouts. And pockets on the glove hold three removable weights (one-third pound each) on the back

A Sample Water Healing
Workout for Knee Injury

A UCLA volleyball player experienced pain every time she bent her knees, so her first Water Healing Workout was built from deep-water, straight-leg exercises only. The quad stretch was the only bent-knee exercise that didn't cause her pain. Over time, however, she was able to add many of the other bent-knee exercises.

She warmed up with deep-water walking, then stretched. The fitness portion of her workout came from Deep Waterpower, Level 2, then 3. Next she did the Specific Rehab Exercises (SREs) for knees, then at the end of each Water Healing Workout she practiced volleyball blocks, still in deep water.

Because her lower-body exercises were limited, she put extra energy into her upper-body work in order to elevate her heart rate and retain fitness. She wore Speedo Aquatic SwimMitt XTs (see description on page 101) during the arm exercises and the water-walking intervals to increase resistance. During intervals, she could choose to concentrate on speed or power. For speed, she turned her hands to slice through the water and avoid the resistance. But when she wanted to concentrate on power, she turned her hands so the webbing caught more water and forced her arms, shoulders, chest, and back to work harder.

Each week, the athlete tried all the Deep Waterpower exercises again. When she could begin slow, gentle bending of the knee, she added water running to her interval training. The walking was her intensive work period, while the running was her slow recovery period. Every week, she tried the exercises that had originally caused her pain and added to her workout the ones she could now perform painlessly. With the new exercises she always started slowly, moving through her full range of motion. Several weeks later she began to add speed.

The front and back flutter kicks caused the athlete pain throughout her program, probably because she was an excellent swimmer and kicked so powerfully. Those two exercises never were added to her program, but she worked all the others into her routine over four weeks time.

At the end of each session, the athlete stretched again, then iced both of her knees for fifteen minutes.

The Athlete's Deep Waterpower Exercises

First Selection Process, nineteen of twenty-eight selected

Water Walking (Exercise 2, page 90)

Water Walking Intervals, no running (Exercise 3, page 92)

Straight-Leg Twist (Exercise 5, page 95)

The
Complete
Waterpower
Workout
Book

232

Quick Scissors (Exercise 7, page 97)

Water Walking Intervals, no running (Exercise 8, page 98)

Abdominals on Bodyciser (see Photo 35, page 325)

Flies (Exercise 10, page 101)

V Kicks (Exercise 11, page 102)

Back Kicks (Exercise 12, page 103)

Water Walking Intervals, no running (Exercise 13, page 104)

Up/Down Pull (Exercise 14, page 105)

Dig Deep (Exercise 15, page 106)

Arm Curls (Exercise 16, page 107)

Straight-Leg Deep Kick (Exercise 19, page 109)

Scissors (Exercise 22, page 111)

Pendulum (Exercise 23, page 112)

Dips (Exercise 24, page 113)

Quad Stretch (Exercise 25, page 114)

Hamstring Stretch (Exercise 26, page 115)

Second Selection Process one week later, twenty-two of twenty-eight exercises
She added the following to her existing program, placed in the appropriate numerical order:

Water Running (Exercise 1, page 88)

Intervals (slow running during recovery period, Exercise 3, page 92)

Curl and Stretch (Exercise 27, page 116)

Body Swing (Exercise 28, page 117)

Third Selection Process one week later, twenty-five of twenty-eight exercises
Add in appropriate numerical order:

Bent-Knee Twist (Exercise 4, page 94)

Bicycling (Exercise 18, page 108)

Fourth Selection Process one week later, twenty-six of twenty-eight exercises
Add in appropriate numerical order:

Heel Lifts (Exercise 6, page 96)

Once the UCLA athlete's knees could tolerate some gentle weight bearing, she introduced some Waterpower Warm-Down exercises, then eventually Waterpower Workout exercises. Before returning to the court for practice, she tested her knees with a strenuous Twenty-five-Minute Powerhouse Workout.

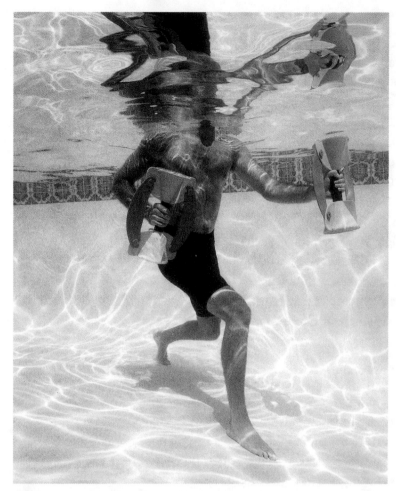

SpaBells with Power Vanes provide extra resistance for upper body exercise.

of the hand. This capacity for adding and removing weight makes the glove valuable as a progressive resistance tool in the rehabilitation of wrists, elbows, arms, and shoulders. The XT in the name stands for cross training, for this glove is also a staple of fitness swimmers. (See photo G, page 195.)

Water Wafer. The Water Wafer is a bright blue foam circle twelve inches in diameter. You can draw it through the water for upper-body strengthening, or stand on it. Standing on this small piece with no edges requires good balance, but also provides a minimal closed-kinetic chain for knee, hip, and ankle rehab (see Photo 19C, page 319).

Specific Rehabilitation Exercises for the Lower Body

You've learned in Chapter 8 that there are many possible components in a Water Healing Workout: (1) Deep-Water Running and Walking Warm-Up, (2) Stretching, (3) Deep-Water Intervals, (4) The Deep Waterpower Workout, (5) The Waterpower Warm-Down, (6) The Waterpower Workout, (7) Twenty-Five-Minute Powerhouse Workout, (8) Gait Training, (9) Specific Rehabilitation Exercises (SREs), (10) Resistance Training, and (11) Sport-Specific or Dance-Specific Waterpower Workouts. After **diagnosis and consultation with your doctor or physical therapist,** use the chart below to know which components to include during each phase of your rehabilitation.

You've chosen your exercises from several of these components and written them on a list that will accompany you each time you go to the pool.

Now complete your list of exercises by finding your injury here in this chapter on lower-body injuries or in the next on upper-body injuries and then adding specific rehab exercises (SREs) for that injured part of your body to your workout.

Water Healing Workout Components
for Nonsurgical Lower-Body Injuries

Exception: Those with grade III sprains (complete tears) of anterior cruciate, posterior cruciate, medial collateral, and lateral collateral ligaments should treat their injury as though it had been surgically repaired. See major knee surgery, page 314.

Phase 1

1. Deep-Water Running or Walking Warm-Up
2. Stretching
3. The Deep Waterpower Workout, Level 1 or 2, depending on fitness level
   If the injury site is your knee:
   Do the straight-leg Water Walking intervals only
   Do not bend the knee to do Water Running
4. Gait Training, with flotation belt
   Exercises 24 and 25 only (pages 264 and 265)
5. Specific Rehabilitation Exercises (SREs)—braced if needed to avoid pain
   Two sets of ten reps
6. Stretching
7. **ICE**

Phase 2

1. Deep-Water Running and Walking Warm-Up
2. Stretching
3. The Deep Waterpower Workout, Level 1, 2, or 3, with walking and running intervals
4. Gait Training, with flotation belt
   Exercises 24, 25, and 26 only (pages 264 through 266).

The
Complete
Waterpower
Workout
Book

236

5. SREs, adding speed as tolerated—braced if needed to avoid pain

   Three sets of ten reps
6. Stretching
7. **ICE**

Phase 3

1. Deep-Water Running and Walking Warm-Up
2. Stretching
3. The Waterpower Warm-Down, progressing to The Waterpower Workout, Level 1, 2, or 3, depending on fitness level
4. Sport-Specific or Dance-Specific Waterpower Workout (optional)
5. SREs, add resistance equipment

   Three sets of twenty reps
6. Stretching
7. **ICE**

Phase 4

1. Deep-Water Running and Walking Warm-Up
2. Stretching
3. The Waterpower Workout, progressing up to Level 3, then The Twenty-five-Minute Powerhouse Workout
4. Sport-Specific or Dance-Specific Waterpower Workout (optional)
5. SREs with resistance and speed

   Four sets of twenty reps
6. Stretching
7. **ICE**

Foot, Ankle, Lower Leg

The foot is composed of twenty-six bones loosely connected to allow for maximum flexibility in movement. During weight bearing the arch of the foot rocks inward, making it flexible and able to adapt to terrain. This is called pronation. During the push-off phase of the walking or running stride, the joint structure within the foot also allows for an outward rocking of the foot bones to a locked position, providing a rigid lever for propulsion. This is called supination.

The foot connects to the leg at the ankle joint. This joint is fairly well protected by ligaments; it allows the foot to move primarily upward and downward. Side to side movements primarily occur in smaller joints below the ankle.

The lower leg has two long bones. The larger weight-bearing bone of the shin is called the tibia. The lower end of this bone is your inner anklebone. The smaller bone on the outside of the leg is the fibula. The bottom of the fibula is your outer anklebone.

Most of the muscles that move the foot and ankle are attached at one end to the tibia or fibula and at the other end to the various bones of the foot. When you are rehabilitating a foot or ankle injury, concentrate on exercises that build strength in the muscles of the shin and calf.

COMMON INJURIES OF THE FOOT, ANKLE, AND LOWER LEG

Plantar fasciitis is an inflammation of the broad band of connective tissue (fascia) located at the bottom of the foot that extends from the heel to the base of the toes. Pain is felt on the sole of the foot, in the arch, or near the heel. A **neuroma** is an inflammation of a nerve ending located between the long bones of the foot near the toes. You might feel pain from a neuroma in the ball of the foot in the area between the toes. **Fractures** and **stress fractures** can occur in the bones of the foot, ankle, or shin. A fracture is a traumatic forceful breaking of a bone while a stress fracture occurs from the accumulation of repetitive micro stresses.

A **sprained ankle** occurs when the foot is forcibly turned inward or outward, damaging the ligaments that hold the foot to the leg. Pain and swelling occur immediately and range of motion becomes limited.

A **shin splint** is an inflammation in the lower leg of a muscle, tendon, or bone, or any combination of these three. Muscles can be torn or strained in the lower leg either from a one-time traumatic incident or they can break down from repetitive stress. Similarly, the tendons that connect the lower leg muscles to the tibia, fibula, and foot can be strained either traumatically or over time. Regardless of how tendons are strained, the resulting inflammation is called **tendinitis.** The Achilles tendon is a cordlike tendon that attaches the large calf muscles to the heel bone. Inflammation of this tendon—Achilles tendinitis—is perhaps the most common and disabling of lower-leg tendon problems.

Fractures are usually cast for several weeks to several months. Begin suspended Water Healing Workouts in your waterproof cast. When it is removed, you can begin your

The
Complete
Waterpower
Workout
Book

238

SREs. Stress fractures do not require a cast, but the injured area should be immobilized for several weeks. Get your doctor's approval before beginning a Water Healing Workout.

Acute injuries to the ankle, foot, and lower leg require the elimination of weight bearing, so you will perform The Deep Waterpower Workout exercises until you can begin to touch lightly down on the pool bottom while continuing to wear your flotation device.

Specific Rehabilitation Exercises 1 through 6 will help in the rehabilitation of all the aforementioned injuries. While exercises 5 and 6 require full entry to the pool, exercises 1 through 4 can be done sitting on a step or the side of the pool, or even at home in your bathtub on days you can't make it to the pool. At home, use *only* cold or ice water (under 60 degrees) during Phase 1 of your rehab. From Phase 2 on, do the exercises in hot water (100 to 105 degrees) first, then repeat them in cold.

Because movement of your leg through water causes passive movement of the foot, you should **tape, splint, or otherwise brace a sprained ankle, torn Achilles tendon, or plantar fasciitis before entering the water.** Once the workout portion of the session is complete, you can remove the tape or splint to begin regaining strength and function as you do the SREs.

When you have worked your way to Phase 3 (see pages 223 and 224), add a swim fin to increase resistance in exercises 1 through 4.

Do the exercises that follow with your healthy foot first. In this way, you can master the coordination of the exercise without any pain, then apply that learning to your injured foot. Note the difference in range of motion between the healthy and the injured foot. This difference will decrease over time. Once you have learned the exercises, perform them only with the affected foot.

Exercise 1. Ankle Flexion and Extension
Ankle flexors and extensors

Sit on a step or ledge with your healthy leg straight in front of you. Point your healthy foot toward the bottom of the pool (Photo 1A), then back toward the surface (Photo 1B). Notice how far the foot moves in each direction. Then begin slowly to move your injured foot toward the bottom of the pool, then back toward the surface. Reach to the point in your range of motion where you first feel pain. Back off slightly and **do your subsequent repetitions only within that pain-free range.**

1A

1B

The
Complete
Waterpower
Workout
Book

240

Exercise 2. Foot Inversion and Eversion

Ankle invertors, ankle evertors

Stay on the step or ledge with your straight healthy leg forward. Hold the hip, knee, and lower leg stationary. Move only the foot from side to side, reaching to the position shown in Photo 2A, then in Photo 2B.

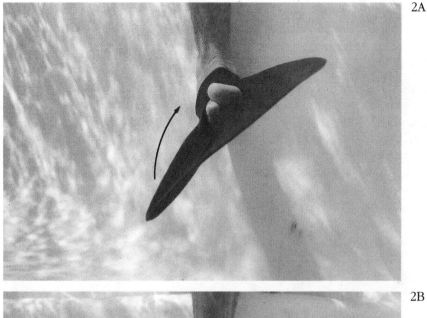

2A

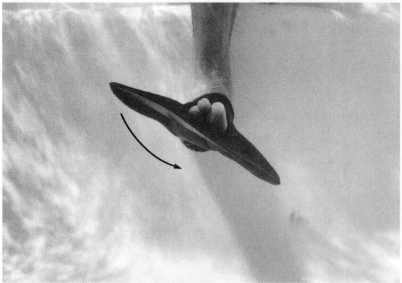

2B

Fins are added to exercises 1 through 4 when you reach Phase 3 of your rehabilitation.

Exercise 3. Foot Circles
Ankle flexors, extensors, evertors, invertors

Circle your healthy foot using your big toe to trace the numbers of the clock. Hold the leg motionless and move only the foot. Circle the same foot counterclockwise. Once you learn the movement, *slowly* perform clockwise and counterclockwise circles with your injured foot for the number of reps shown in the chart, pages 236–237.

Exercise 4. Write with Big Toe
Ankle flexors, extensors, evertors, invertors

Hold the lower leg of your healthy foot motionless as you "write" your phone number using your big toe as the "pen." Once you get the idea, slowly begin again with your injured foot. Write your address, then the names of your favorite cities or countries. Instead of counting reps (because you can't count and spell at the same time), write for two thirty-second periods in Phase 1, three thirty-second periods in Phase 2, three one-minute periods in Phase 3, and four one-minute periods in Phase 4.

The
Complete
Waterpower
Workout
Book

242

Exercise 5. Toe Raises
Ankle flexors

Stand erect in chest-deep water facing the side of the pool. Place both hands on the side of the pool for balance. Slowly lift your heels to stand on your toes, then slowly return your heels to the pool bottom. At Phase 3, advance to single-leg toe raises, but perform only the Phase 1 sets and reps: two sets of ten reps. Work your way gradually back to Phase 3 reps and sets. Most pools have a downhill slope in the shallow end. During phases 1 and 2 of your rehab, perform exercises 5 and 6 with your toes facing downhill. During phases 3 and 4, face your toes uphill to increase the stretch and workload.

5

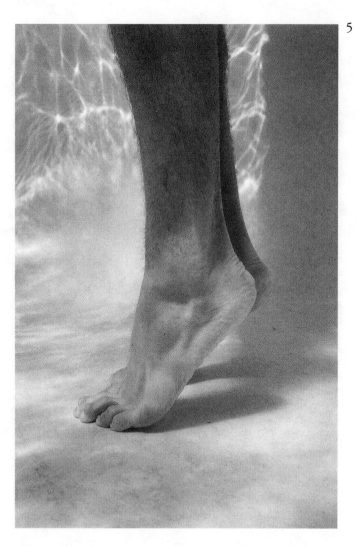

Exercise 6. Negative Toe Raises
Ankle flexors

Stand on the edge of a step that allows you to be in crotch-deep water or deeper. If your lowest available step forces you into mid-thigh or knee-deep water, skip this exercise. Lower your heels below the level of the step to the position shown in Photo 6A. Now lift your heels to stand on your toes (Photo 6B) and return to the starting position. When you have progressed to three sets of twenty reps in Phase 3, execute single-leg negative toe raises, starting first with ten reps on the healthy foot, then repeating ten reps with the injured foot. In Phase 4 work your way up the steps to shallower and shallower water.

6A

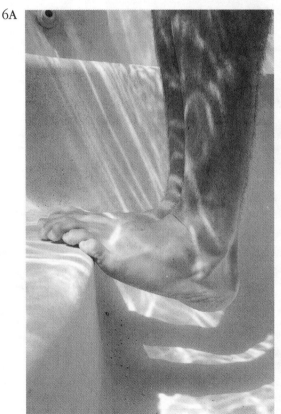
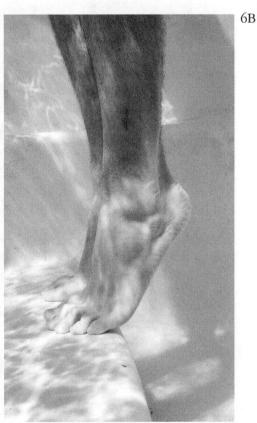

6B

The
Complete
Waterpower
Workout
Book

244

Knee

The knee joint consists of three bones—the femur (large thigh bone), the tibia (shin bone), and a small, free-floating bone called the patella (kneecap). The femur and the tibia meet to form a hinge joint and are held together by the ligaments (medial and lateral collateral, anterior and posterior cruciate) and the joint capsule that surrounds the joint. Injuries to these structures are known as sprains. When a ligament is injured, early-controlled motion can speed its healing. Complete tears of ligaments, however, require a period of immobilization and a doctor's release to begin exercise.

The patella is lodged in the quadricep tendon. Most problems involving the patella are thought to be caused by improper "tracking" (up-down gliding) of the patella in the groove on the front of the femur. Balanced quadricep strength promotes correct tracking of the patella. An imbalance in muscle strength causes improper tracking that will damage the surfaces of the femur and the patella. This degenerative condition is referred to as **chondromalacia.** Other problems involving the patella include inflammation of the quadriceps tendon that houses it. Such **patella tendinitis** can be either above or below the kneecap. Balanced muscle strength and good flexibility remedies all of the above conditions.

The iliotibial band is a wide band of connective tissue located on the outside of the thigh extending from the hip to the knee. Imbalance in the alignment of the pelvis or discrepancy in leg length causes altered function of this band at the knee. This in turn causes friction and painful irritation on the outside of the knee. To improve this condition, you must stretch and strengthen the large thigh and hip muscles and correct the mechanics of the pelvis.

In its bony design, the knee joint is inherently unstable; therefore it relies heavily on the ligaments and musculature for stability. When injury occurs to any structure in the knee, pain inhibits full movement or function. The large muscles of your thighs—quadriceps and hamstrings—immediately begin to weaken and atrophy. This weakness of the muscles allows strain on the injured structure, which causes more pain and thus more weakness: This downward cycle continues until you interrupt it by strengthening the muscles to take the impact off the injured structures of the joint. By performing your rehabilitative exercises in water, you can more easily select the appropriate amount of stress to strengthen the muscles and halt this downward cycle, which starts you back toward function and fitness.

Arthritic conditions of the knee are common, especially in older people. **Degenerative osteoarthritis** is an inflammation of the cartilage that covers the ends of the bones that meet at a joint. It is a painful condition characterized by swelling that limits range of motion and causes loss of strength in the surrounding muscles.

Because weight bearing on an injured or arthritic knee is painful, you will start with The Deep Waterpower Workout for the fitness portion of your program. Exercises in water should begin even before you can bend your knee. Remember that you can do water walking and all the straight-legged exercises, which strengthen the thighs.

Exercises 7 through 9, below, help rehabilitate the most common knee injuries addressed above. (Remember that these are nonsurgical knee conditions. If surgery was recommended for your knee, but you chose nonsurgical therapy, or if you have had recent surgical repair, see Chapter 11.) For an even more thorough rehabilitation of your knee, also do the SREs, exercises 10 through 15 on page 250 under Hips, Buttocks, and Thighs. If the pain is severe, wear a waterproof brace into the water to protect your knee. The brace protects your injury so you can train harder during the fitness portion of your Water Healing Workout. In Phase 1, continue to wear the brace even as you do the specific rehab exercises. During Phase 2, you can gently attempt the SREs without the brace, but replace it if you experience undue pain. From Phase 3 on, you should be able to perform the rehab work without the brace and without pain.

Avoid or be particularly cautious with these Deep Waterpower exercises:

Heel Lifts (Exercise 6, page 96)
Quick Scissors (Exercise 7, page 97)
Flies (Exercise 10, page 101)
Kicking exercises (17–21, pages 108 to 110)
Quad Stretch (Exercise 25, page 114)
Curl and Stretch (Exercise 27, page 116)
Body Swing (Exercise 28, page 117)

The
Complete
Waterpower
Workout
Book

246

Exercise 7. Quad Extensions
Quads, hamstrings, hip flexors

During phases 1 and 2, perform Exercise 34 in its usual way as shown on page 71. During Phase 3, add the Hydro-Tone boot to your foot and slowly try this exercise. If you experience pain, take the boot off and wait another week to try again. If you are able to make this movement without pain, place your hand on your thigh just above your knee (Photo 7) to stabilize your leg against the powerful resistance you will encounter wearing the boot.

In Phase 4, continue wearing the boot and gradually add speed.

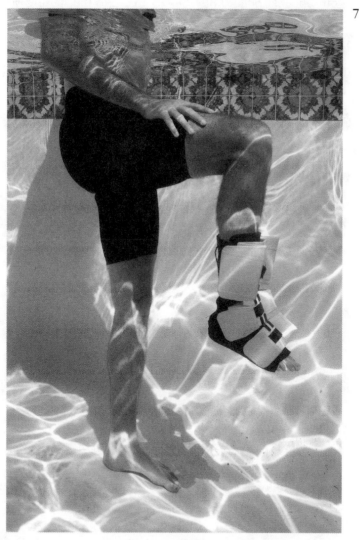

7

When using a Hydro-Tone boot, stabilize the position of your knee by placing your hand on your thigh.

Exercise 8. Hamstring Curls

Hamstrings, quads, gastrocnemius

During Phases 1 and 2, perform Exercise 35 (page 72) as usual. During Phase 3, add a Hydro-Tone boot and slowly follow the directions below. This slight modification in stance allows for best utilization of the extra resistance. If you experience any pain, however, remove the boot and wait another week before trying again.

Face the side of the pool, place both feet several feet away from the side, and brace yourself with both hands as in Photo 8A. Notice the straight line of the body as it leans slightly forward. **Keep your knees together** and slowly raise the foot of your affected knee toward your buttocks (Photo 8B). Slowly return to the starting position.

In Phase 4, continue wearing the boot and gradually add speed.

8A 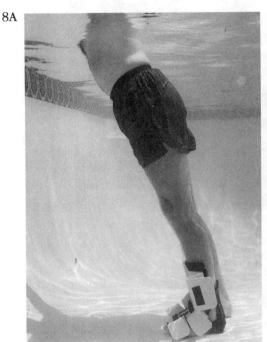 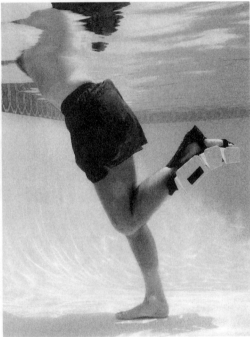 8B

The
Complete
Waterpower
Workout
Book

248

Exercise 9. Bicycling *(Exercise 19, page 56)*

Modify the exercise by keeping your feet below the surface of the water during phases 1 and 2, then begin the full, powerful bicycling motion.

Hips, Buttocks, and Thighs

The hip is where the thigh bone (femur) attaches to the pelvis in a ball-and-socket joint. This joint is extremely strong, and at the same time it offers great range of movement. The muscles located in the buttocks, the pelvis, and the thighs control movement at this joint.

The most common injuries in the hip are **arthritic conditions, tendinitis, bursitis** (inflammation of the fluid sac that prevents friction), **fractures,** and **strains** and **bruises** of the muscles: the three gluteal muscles (maximus, medius, and minimus), hip rotators, and iliopsoas. Injuries of the buttocks and thighs include tendinitis and muscle strains to the gluteals, quadriceps, hamstrings, abductors, and adductors. A muscle strain is damage to a number of muscle fibers. The amount of muscle tissue damaged dictates the degree of the strain. A first-degree strain is the most mild, while a third-degree strain is a complete tear. The result of these muscle injuries is a functional weakness that may be severe in grade II or III injuries or may be subtle and only become apparent with high-intensity performance in grade I strains. The primary goal when rehabilitating muscle tears is to regain full muscular strength and flexibility. The part of the muscle that attaches to a bone is called the tendon. It may be flat or cord-like. Injuries to these structures are called tendinitis, which can be remedied by icing and performing stretching and strengthening exercises.

By starting early-movement water exercises you will experience less atrophy in the involved muscles and less strain on the tendons, while insuring that your body creates a functional scar, not one that will tear again.

If the muscles you strained move the hip joint (hip abductors and adductors, hip flexors, hip rotators, and gluteus maximus), start with exercises 7 and 8, above, that move only the knee. In this way, you keep the surrounding muscles strong while the injured ones heal. Conversely, if you injured the muscles that move the knee (quads, hamstrings), start with exercises 10, 11, and 15 below that move only the hip.

When you begin the exercises that force you to contract the strained or torn muscle, move slowly through a pain-free range of motion. At first you may have only a few inches of motion in each direction. However, if you feel no pain, begin reaching for a wider and still wider range of motion. By Phase 2, when you can work your hip and knee through their full, pain-free range of motion, you can add speed to gain resistance from the water. During Phase 3, you will add resistance equipment as you do your specific rehab exercises.

Perform all these exercises standing poolside holding on to the side of the pool with one hand. Work your noninjured leg first. Then turn 180 degrees to work your injured leg. You will continue to do these SREs on both sides. It's easy to think the supporting leg isn't doing much, but don't underestimate how hard it works to maintain stability for the body. The leg muscles must perform balanced isometric contractions to provide this stability. When you stand on your injured leg to work the healthy leg, be cautious, for the supporting leg *will* be working.

Exercise 10. Lateral Leg Lifts *(Exercise 31, page 67)*

Exercise 11. Leg Circles *(Exercise 32, page 68)*

Exercise 12. Knee Swivels *(Exercise 33, page 70)*

Don't do this exercise if you have had a hip replacement.

Exercise 13. Quad Extensions *(Exercise 34, page 71)*

Exercise 14. Hamstring Curls *(Exercise 35, page 72)*

The
Complete
Waterpower
Workout
Book

250

Exercise 15. Standing Leg Swings
Hip flexors, gluteus maximus, hip adductors, hamstrings

Continue standing erect on the injured leg, working the noninjured leg. Swing your healthy leg straight forward (Photo 15A), then swing it down and to the rear (Photo 15B). Tighten your abdominal and gluteal muscles to help protect your lower back.

15A

15B

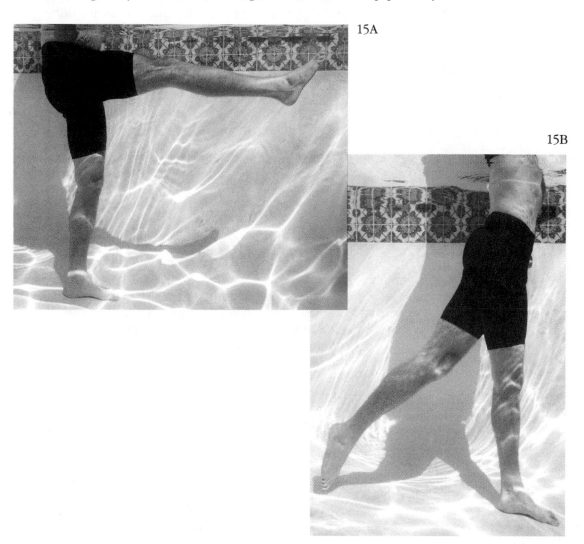

   Now repeat exercises 10 through 15 standing on your healthy leg, working the injured leg. During Phase 3, add a Hydro-Tone boot to the working leg to provide added resistance and induce strength gains. If you only use one boot at a time you will be able to maneuver more easily than if you wear two and often get your boots tangled together. In Phase 4, continue using the added resistance and increase speed as well.

Back

The spinal column consists of twenty-four moving vertebrae—from top to bottom: seven cervical, twelve thoracic, and five lumbar vertebrae, each separated by a fibrocartilage disk. The sacrum and the coccyx are fused vertebrae located at the base of the spine. From the first cervical to the fifth lumbar vertebrae, the bodies of the vertebrae become larger, providing for efficient weight bearing. The spine is a flexible column of these bones and cartilage held together by ligaments, fasciae, and muscle. It can be thought of as a portable tower, with the muscles and fasciae acting as guy wires. This structure allows for tremendous flexibility of movement: forward, backward, side-to-side, and rotation to the right and left.

The spine is at the center of all human movement. The lower extremities are anchored to the spine by way of the pelvis. The upper extremities by way of the shoulder girdles attach to the thorax (rib cage), which attaches to the spine. The head is directly on top of the spine. With its great functional role in human movements of all kinds, the back is susceptible to many varied stresses. It's no wonder eight out of ten Americans experience back pain during their lives. This pain may last only a few days or weeks; but for many, pain continues for months or even years.

Injuries to the spine can involve muscles, fasciae, ligaments, the fibrocartilage disks, or the bony vertebrae themselves. Common back problems fall into three basic categories: (1) postural syndromes, (2) disk injuries, and (3) spinal dysfunction. The cervical and thoracic areas of the spine are particularly sensitive to pain from postural syndromes, while the lumbar area is more likely to suffer from disk injuries. However, dysfunction can occur in any area of the spine.

Postural syndromes result from improper use of the body in activities of daily living such as standing, walking, sitting, lifting, and bending. Commonly, poor posture in youth becomes fixed as poor posture in young adulthood and the years beyond. All connective tissue shortens with time, and if left unstretched, will permanently adapt to the shortened position. Adaptive shortening results in abnormal stress being placed on the various body structures. For example, tight pectoral muscles of the chest cause forward, rounded shoulders, forcing the head to a forward position. Weak muscles also cause postural stress, because they fail to support proper spinal curve alignment. For instance, weak abdominal muscles allow increased lower-back curve. Weak upper-back muscles allow the increased thoracic curve of "dowager's hump."

Disk injuries involve the fibrocartilage shock absorbers between vertebrae. Each disk is composed of a syruplike center (nucleus pulposus) surrounded by concentric layers of cartilage. All of this is wrapped in a ligament called the annulus. Habits such as slouching, sitting for extended periods, or lifting improperly place the lower back in a bent-forward (flexed) position that is contrary to its normal curve. In this flexed position, pressure within the disk increases and places great stress on the back wall of the disk. This area eventually breaks down, allowing the nucleus pulposus to push out of the disk and push on pain-sensitive structures. Pain may be located solely in the back or it may radiate down one leg or the other. Disk injuries can also be caused by one-time, traumatic events such as a motorcycle accident, a football tackle, or a fall.

The
Complete
Waterpower
Workout
Book

252

Treatment of disk injuries has changed dramatically in the past decade. New treatments involve extension exercises. The theory is that if forward bending and excessive flexion to the lumbar spine causes disk injuries, then backward bending or extension of the lumbar spine will help to center the bulging disk and reduce the bulging nucleus pulposus.

Spinal dysfunction occurs as a result of injury to the back. After the injury has healed, the formation of scar tissue in the muscles, fasciae, ligaments, or disk may alter joint function in the spine and cause painful limitations of movement.

The rehabilitation process for all categories must include three important components: (1) **spinal protection,** (2) **therapeutic exercise,** and (3) **ice.** Today's progressive health-care practitioners now ask back-pain patients to become active participants in their own back-care programs by improving their biomechanics, thus protecting their backs from further harm, by improving their strength and flexibility through exercise, and by icing regularly. Patients must move correctly through their daily activities—during sitting, standing, walking, twisting, and bending. Healing can be disrupted from something so simple as one or two improper movements. The therapeutic exercises consist of stretching and strengthening while the back is in a safe position. Stretching in the water provides buoyancy that increases your stability so you can protect your back while you effectively isolate specific muscle groups. The exercises to follow should be done in the sequence shown to achieve the desired results.

Ice has replaced heat as the treatment of choice for back inflammation, swelling, pain, and spasm. Although icing a back injury is uncomfortable for the first few minutes, the back soon becomes numb, and the healing that results is well worth the discomfort. After a few icing sessions, even the initial discomfort will diminish. (See box, page 000.)

Finally, prevent further damage to your back by solving postural problems. Perhaps your biomechanics are precise during your sports activity, but then you become careless with your body once you leave the locker room. Check your sitting position in your car, your chair at work or at home; begin a faithful water stretching and strengthening program; and apply ice frequently and regularly. By doing all three, you can resolve your symptoms in the shortest possible time.

As you perform the exercises that are part of your Water Healing Workout, devote extra time to Waterpower stretching exercises 30 (page 66) and 36 through 38 (pages 73 through 75) and Deep Waterpower Exercise 27 (page 116). Do an extra set of Exercise 9 (Abdominals, page 100) and Exercise 12 (Back Kicks, page 103), which strengthen the abdominals and the buttocks.

Considerable back pain can be avoided when fitness programs are transferred into the water. But during episodes of severe spasm or back pain, it is a good idea to know which of the specific rehab exercises can offer you relief. Once the curling and stretching of Exercise 16 relieves some of your pain, gently try the others. They are "assisted-swimming" exercises designed to get you moving comfortably again while they strengthen your back and abdominal muscles to help you maintain healthy posture and reduce back pain. If traditional swimming has aggravated your back pain in the past, you should find great relief from the precise modifications here. Flotation belts, face masks, and snorkels decompress your lower back and eliminate spinal rotation. And this equipment will help even the weakest swimmer perform all of these exercises.

Exercises 16 through 21, below, can be performed while swimming up and down the pool, but if the pool is small, or if back pain is severe, tether yourself to the side of the pool to eliminate the need to perform the sometimes painful turn at the end of each lap. You will strengthen different muscles swimming face down from those you strengthen when swimming face up, so swim both ways. In the face-down position, use Exercise 17 to prepare you to reach a full crawl in Exercise 18. Exercises 19 and 20 prepare you to swim the full backstroke in Exercise 21. If these swimming exercises are your SREs, you will perform minutes rather than sets and reps. Start with one minute the first time you try each swimming exercise. Add thirty seconds each workout until you have reached five to ten minutes of each stroke.

If you don't swim, and are afraid to try "assisted swimming," skip to exercises 35 and 38 in Chapter 11, in which you will lie on a floating mattress, the Bodyciser, for your back exercises. If your doctor approves spinal extension, stand at the side of the pool and gently try exercises 22 and 23, below.

Avoid or be particularly cautious with these Deep Waterpower (DW) and Waterpower (WP) exercises:

Straight-Leg Twist (DW Exercise 5, page 95)
Back Kicks, (DW Exercise 12, page 103, and WP Exercise 13, page 48)
Slap Kick (DW Exercise 21, page 110, and WP Exercise 24, page 60)
Side-Straddle Jumps (WP Exercise 5, page 40)

Bend your knees slightly if you perform the following:

V Kicks (DW Exercise 11, page 102, and WP Exercise 8, page 43)
Straight-Leg Deep Kick (DW Exercise 19, page 109, and WP Exercise 20, page 57)
Pendulum (DW Exercise 23, page 112, and WP Exercise 22, page 59)
Hamstring Stretch (DW Exercise 26, page 115, and WP Exercise 37, page 74)
Side-Straddle Jumps (WP Exercise 5, page 40)
Leg Swings (WP Exercise 11, page 46)
Front Kicks (WP Exercise 12, page 47)

Put on your face mask for the following exercises and **create a "seal"** so that no water will leak in. Follow these suggestions:

- Pull back all your hair so it won't go under the mask. Hair under the edge of a face mask lets water leak in.

- Men with moustaches should consider trimming the hair down a bit below the nose. The face mask can't establish a good seal on your lip if hair is present.

- Lift the strap high onto the crown of your hair rather than lower, where it has a less efficient angle of pull.

The
Complete
Waterpower
Workout
Book

254

Exercise 16. Kick, Curl, and Stretch with Flotation Belt, Face Mask, and Snorkel

Abdominals, erector spinae, rhomboids, trapezius, hip flexors, gluteus maximus, hip adductors, hamstrings, quads

Strap a flotation belt around your hips and turn the buckle to the center of your back. This placement gives you the most lift from your belt. As you step into the water, the belt will naturally want to rise to the surface, so wait until you lie flat on the water surface, then breathe through the snorkel and pull the belt down to your hips. Keep your arms at your sides and gently kick at least ten yards (Photo 16A), then curl up into a ball (Photo 16B). Take five to ten slow, deep breaths as you relax your back muscles. Then gently stretch your feet and hands away from each other on the surface of the water (Photo 16C). Your arms return to your sides as you go through the cycle again: kick, curl, stretch. Repeat five times or until you experience relief. If you find your snorkel slips under the water as you curl, you may have to ask a friend to hold the snorkel above the water line while you relax and breathe.

16A

16C

16B

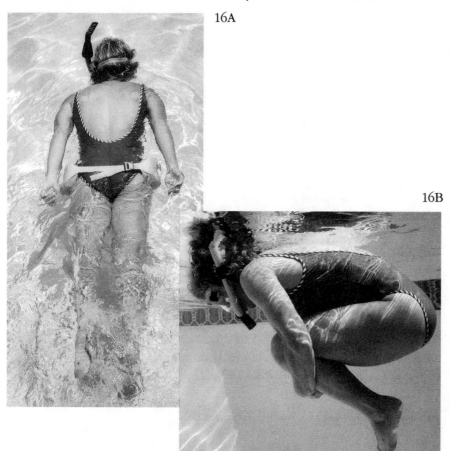

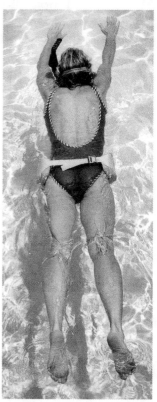

Exercise 17. Combined Stroke with Face Mask and Flotation Belt

Gluteus maximus, erector spinae, hip flexors, abdominals, quads, lats, pecs, rhomboids, deltoids, biceps, triceps, wrist flexors and extensors, hip adductors

Seal your face mask onto your face and breathe through your snorkel as you again pull your belt back to your hips. Begin a continuous, alternating up-and-down flutter kick with the legs. The action originates at the hips with the legs kept nearly straight. Gently begin moving your arms through the motion of the breaststroke: Both hands reach straight forward, then they press sideways and downward until they are even with the shoulders (Photo 17). They recover by extending to their forward starting position. Keep on with this for three to five minutes. If you are tethered, be prepared to experience a "pull back" from the tether. Each time you breaststroke, you will move away from the side of the pool, then on the recovery of the arms, the tether will pull you back.

Perform Exercise 17 during several workouts before trying Exercise 18. The crawl requires powerful contractions of the back muscles, so **Exercise 18 should not be attempted while you are still in acute pain or spasm.**

17

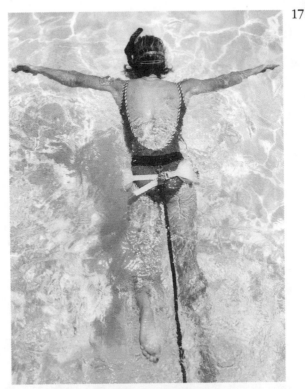

If your pool is small or your back pain severe, tether yourself to the side of the pool to eliminate painful turns at the end of each lap.

The
Complete
Waterpower
Workout
Book

256

Exercise 18. Crawl with Face Mask and Flotation Belt

Trapezius, erector spinae, rhomboids, lats, pecs, deltoids, biceps, triceps, wrist flexors and extensors, hip flexors, gluteus maximus, hip adductors, quads, hamstrings, foot flexors and extensors

Warm up for this exercise with at least three to five minutes of the combined stroke in Exercise 17. Stop and stretch poolside (Exercise 27, page 116), then once again seal your face mask, breathe through the snorkel, and pull your flotation belt into place around your hips. Slowly begin to swim the crawl. If you feel any spasms in your back muscles, stop and return to Exercise 17 for another week. If you feel fine, continue for only two minutes the first time. Add thirty seconds or one minute each workout until you reach ten minutes.

Breathing on only one side develops only one side of the back, causing an imbalance. If you do not know how to breathe on alternating sides, continue to use the face mask to insure equal strengthening of both sides of the back.

18

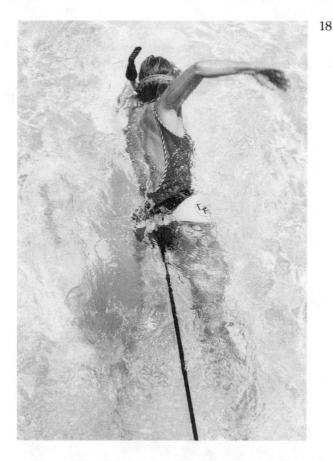

If you feel a strain in your neck during exercises 19, 20, and 21 place another flotation belt or an inflatable cushion under your neck (see Photo 19).

Exercise 19. Combined Stroke on Back with Flotation Belt

Deltoids, lats, trapezius, biceps, triceps, hip flexors, gluteus maximus, hamstrings, quads, hip adductors

Remove the face mask and turn your flotation belt so the buckle is in the front and its major buoyancy power is now at the back of your hips. Lie back on the surface of the water, pull the belt down to your hips, and gently flutter kick. Add the elementary backstroke arms: (1) slide your hands up the side of your body to the armpits; (2) then with the fingers leading, extend the arms fully to the sides, hands level with the top of the head; (3) press the hands and arms toward the feet in a broad sweeping action, parallel to the surface of the water, returning to the starting position. Continue for three to five minutes.

You may feel the urge to do a "frog kick" to match the arm action. **Avoid that movement, because it places undue stress on the back.**

19

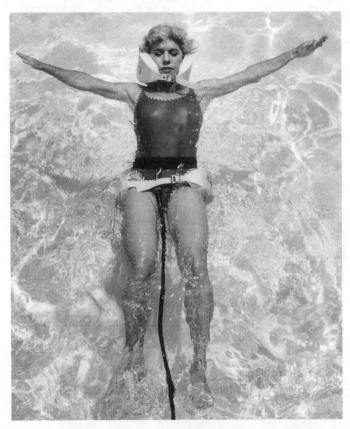

The
Complete
Waterpower
Workout
Book

258

Exercise 20. Modified Backstroke with Flotation Belt

Trapezius, deltoids, lats, wrist flexors and extensors, hip flexors, gluteus maximus, hip adductors, hamstrings, quads, foot flexors and extensors

This is the transition exercise that will prepare you to swim the traditional backstroke. It begins the alternating arm action, but takes your arms through a narrower range of motion and places less force on your back and shoulders than the full backstroke.

Master the arm movements standing up in the shallow end of the pool before trying to perform them while also flutter kicking. Pull the right elbow back as though hitting someone behind you in the chest (Photo 20A). Pause there momentarily, then swing your right hand and forearm toward the water (Photo 20B). Finally, pull your right arm next to your right thigh. Repeat with the left arm, first pulling the elbow back, pausing, then swinging the hand around. Perform this motion several times until you feel it become consistent with both arms. Now lie back in the water, pull your flotation belt down around your hips, and begin to flutter kick. Once you are kicking, add the modified arm stroke. Continue for three to five minutes.

20A 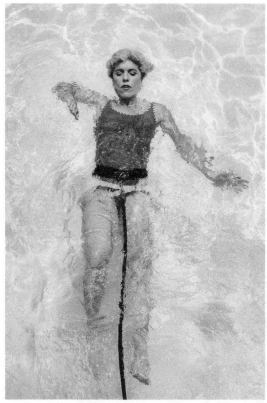 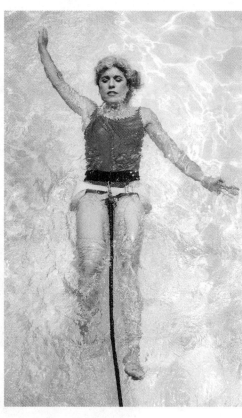 20B

Don't try Exercise 21 until you have mastered 20 and have performed several workouts using the modified stroke without experiencing pain.

Exercise 21. Backstroke with Flotation Belt
Trapezius, deltoids, lats, erector spinae, pecs, hip flexors, gluteus maximus, hip adductors, hamstrings, quads, foot flexors and extensors

Pull your flotation belt around your hips, lie back, and gently begin to flutter kick. Slowly and carefully add the arms. **When you add the full arm stroke, protect your back by softening your kick.** Monitor your body carefully as you perform a full backstroke: (1) the arms are in constant opposition to each other; that is, one arm begins its propulsive action in the water at the same time as the other arm is beginning its recovery action out of the water; (2) as each arm prepares to enter the water, the entire body rolls slightly to the entry side; (3) the arm rotates so that the little finger enters the water first. (See Photo 21.) Start with only a two-minute back crawl. Add thirty seconds at each workout until you work up to ten minutes.

21

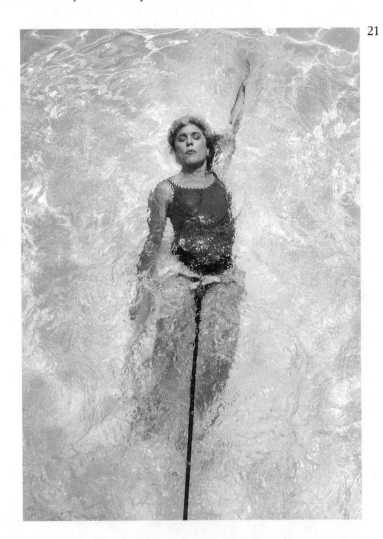

The
Complete
Waterpower
Workout
Book

260

Exercises 22 and 23 should be attempted slowly and cautiously *if* your doctor or physical therapist permits. These two exercises are not designed to stretch or strengthen specific muscles. Rather, they promote proper alignment of the intervertebral disk. If your exercise routine doesn't normally include any backward-bending exercises, be prepared to feel stiffness in the lower back. If you feel any pain, eliminate these exercises from your program.

Exercise 22. Passive Back Extension

Stand poolside with your arms straight, your hands braced against the side of the pool. Maintain an erect posture and keep your heels on the pool bottom as you move your hips forward to the position shown in Photo 22. Hold for a beat, then return to the starting position. Repeat ten times, following the rhythm of the commands: "Pressure ON, Pressure OFF."

22

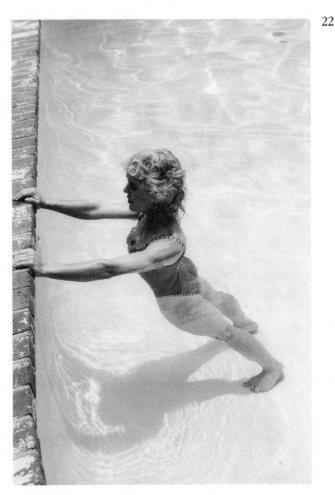

Exercise 23. Crescent Moon

If your back injury is primarily on one side of your back, place that foot forward as you do this next exercise. Then cautiously repeat with the other leg forward.

Stand in a forward stride position, your front knee bent to 90 degrees. Lift your arms straight up overhead. Breathe deeply and reach toward the ceiling. After several breaths, arch slowly back to position 23, chin lifted.

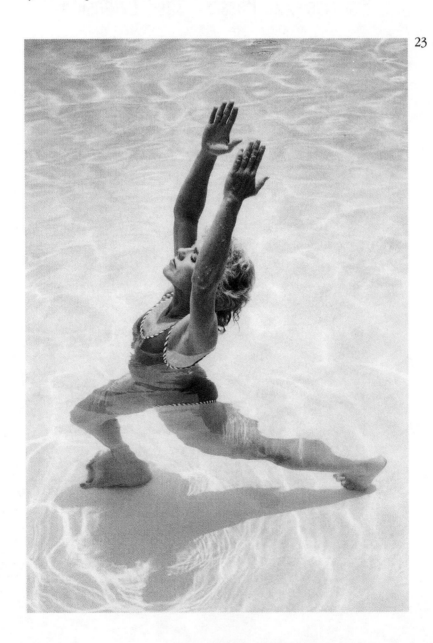

23

The
Complete
Waterpower
Workout
Book

262

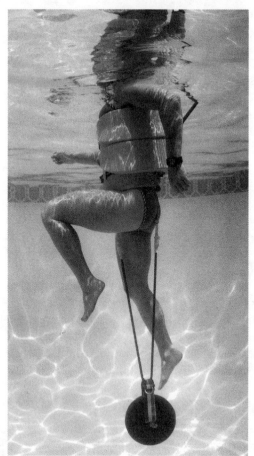

A

A promising form of therapy for backs is floating traction. It must be performed only with the supervision of a doctor or physical therapist.

Gait Training

A debilitating injury may put you on crutches or in a wheelchair for weeks or even months. Even a simple ankle sprain can force you into a limp. By the time you are ready to begin full weight bearing on land, your neuromuscular pattern for walking may have become seriously rusty. In fact, your basic habitual walking pattern may have become a limp. Even your deep-water walking hasn't fully prepared your lower body to handle the landing, transfer of weight, and push-off of walking. But if you practice walking smoothly and symmetrically in chest- to waist-deep water, you can reestablish a correct gait pattern during your convalescence. And by progressing to a marching motion in Exercise 25, you come closer to running. By adding bouncing in Exercise 26, then bounding in 27, you toughen your weight-bearing joints for any unforeseen misstep, thus protecting against reinjury. Wear a flotation device at first to give you increased buoyancy. Remove the device when you feel confident enough to try the exercises without it. **Emphasize opposition of arms and legs to fully regain your coordination.** (See page 11 for a complete explanation.) If you add aqua shoes as in the following photos, you will have better traction as you perform your gait-training exercise.

Exercise 24. Shallow-Water Walking—Forward, Backward, Sideways

Gastroc/soleus complex, tibialis anterior, quads, hamstrings, hip flexors, gluteus maximus, deltoids, pecs, trapezius, rhomboids, teres major, hip adductors and abductors

Stand in chest-deep water with your healthy leg supporting you and your weakened leg in front as you prepare to take the first small step onto it. Hold the opposite arm forward for balance. Swing your arms forcefully through the water as you take first one small step, then another. This arm action helps force your legs into equal and opposite action. Walk slowly across the pool, turn, and walk back. As you repeat this several times, you should start to remember your former walking pattern. Keep the steps short until you can walk without a limp, and then gradually lengthen them.

Walk backward across the pool several times without worrying about your arms. Do, however, look first to make sure you have an unobstructed space behind you. Next try walking sideways with your arms out to the sides for balance. Push off with the healthy leg, step onto the injured leg (Photo 24A), then pull the healthy leg to meet the injured one (Photo 24B). Side step in this manner across the pool, and **keep facing in the same direction** so as you return you will this time push off with the injured leg.

24A

24B

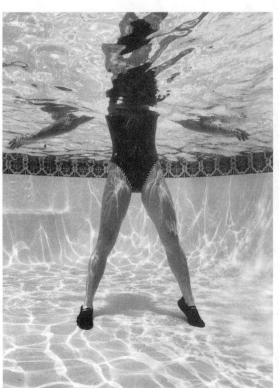
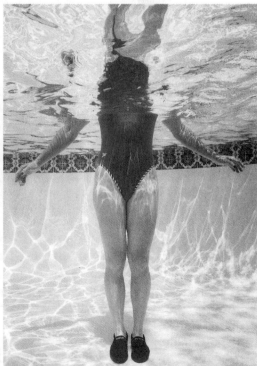

Exercise 25. Marching

Hip flexors, gluteus maximus, sartorius, quads, hamstrings, hip adductors,
gastroc/soleus complex, pecs, rhomboids, biceps

Bend the knee of your injured leg and assume the position shown in Photo 25A. Lean forward and take a step, then lift the other knee up to a similar position. Use bent arms in opposition to the bent knees. March back and forth across the pool several times. When you have been able to perform this, begin lifting up onto the balls of your feet at the push-off of each step (Photo 25B).

25A

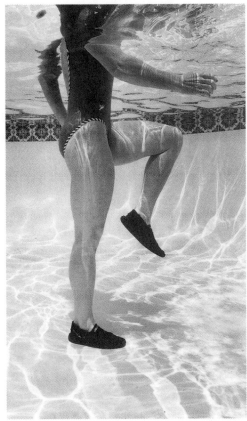

25B

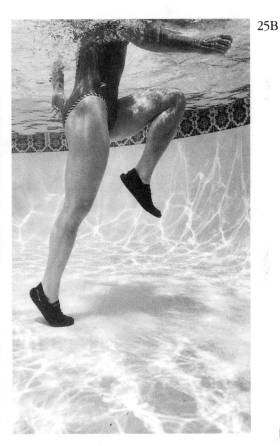

Exercise 26. Bouncing—Front, Back

Quads, hamstrings, gluteus maximus, hip flexors, gastroc/soleus complex, hip adductors

Bend both knees and lower yourself to a half-squat position. Gently and carefully straighten both legs at the same time and jump forward. Immediately bend both knees again, as you smoothly continue this bouncing motion across the pool. After you have bounced forward across the pool several times, bounce backward several times more. When you feel ready, try bouncing forward and backward on only one leg. Try the healthy leg first, then gently try the healing one. If you feel pain simply lift the leg and let the water catch you. Increase the height of your bounces in phases 3 and 4.

Exercise 27. Bounding

Hip flexors, gastroc/soleus complex, sartorius, gluteus maximus, quads, hamstrings, hip adductors, deltoids, pecs, rhomboids, biceps

This is the most advanced of the gait-training exercises and is used primarily in the rehabilitation of athletes. Either skip this one or at least don't try it until exercises 24 through 26 have become easy to do.

Stand on both feet with your weight evenly distributed between them. Simultaneously drive your left knee forward and up and your bent right arm up to the position shown in Photo 27. You must push forcefully with your right leg and foot to gain height away from the pool bottom. Once you have pushed off, **keep your push-off leg straight** and strive for as much "hangtime" in this position as possible. When your left foot touches down, immediately push off into the next bound with your right knee and left arm forward.

The
Complete
Waterpower
Workout
Book

266

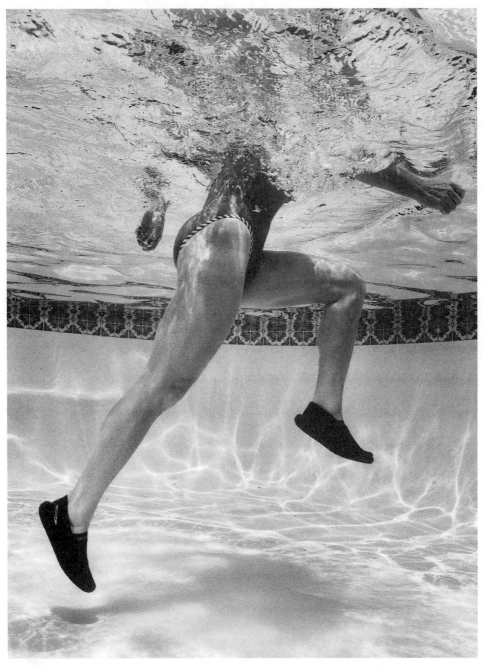

Specific
Rehabilitation
Exercises for
the Lower Body

If your injury did not appear in these pages, it will be in the next chapter.

Specific Rehab Exercises: Lower Body

See chart on pages 236 and 237 for numbers of sets and reps.

Foot, Ankle, and Lower Leg

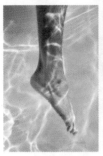 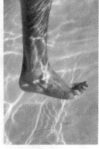

1. Ankle Flexion and Extension

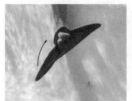 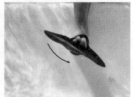

2. Foot Inversion and Eversion

3. Foot Circles
4. Write with Big Toe

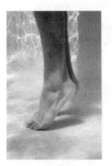

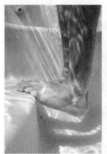 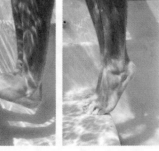

5. Toe Raises

6. Negative Toe Raises

Knee

The
Complete
Waterpower
Workout
Book

268

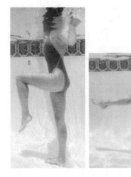

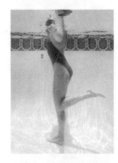

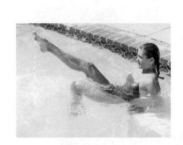

7. Quad Extensions

8. Hamstring Curls

9. Bicycling

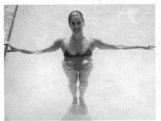
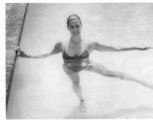

10. Lateral Leg Raises

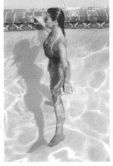
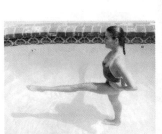
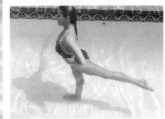

11. Leg Circles

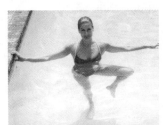
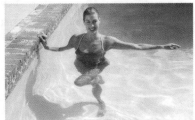

12. Knee Swivels

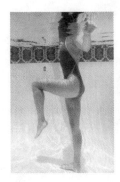
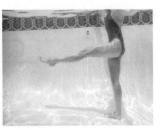
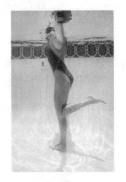

13. Quad Extensions

14. Hamstring Curls

Specific
Rehabilitation
Exercises for
the Lower Body

269

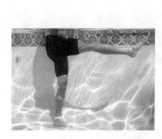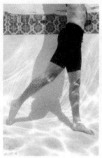

15. Standing Leg Swings

Back

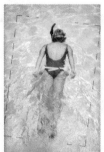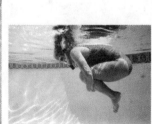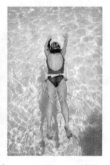

16. Kick, Curl, and Stretch with
Flotation Belt, Face Mask, and Snorkel

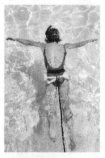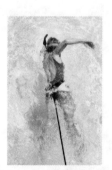

17. Combined Stroke with Flotation Belt,
Face Mask, and Snorkel

18. Crawl with Flotation Belt, Face
Mask, and Snorkel

The
Complete
Waterpower
Workout
Book

270

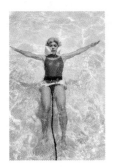

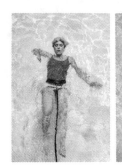

19. Combined Stroke on back with Flotation Belt

20. Modified Backstroke with Flotation Belt

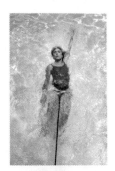

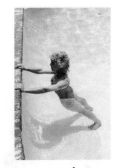

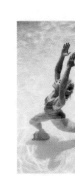

21. Backstroke with Flotation Belt

22. Passive Back Extension

23. Crescent Moon

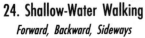

Gait Training

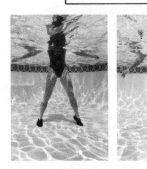

24. Shallow-Water Walking
Forward, Backward, Sideways

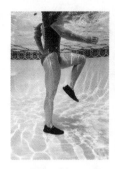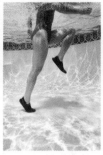

25. Marching, then marching and lift
on toe

26. Bouncing
Forward, Backward, 2 legs, 1 leg

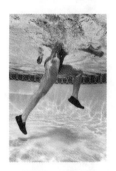

27. Bounding

The
Complete
Waterpower
Workout
Book

272

T e n

Specific
Rehabilitation Exercises
for the Upper Body

A fter diagnosis and consultation with your doctor or physical therapist, find your injury among the injuries to the upper body described below and read your specific rehabilitation exercises. They will be the work you do when you come to the item called SREs in your list of possible components for a Water Healing Workout: (1) Shallow- and Deep-Water Running and Walking Warm-Up, (2) Stretching, (3) Deep-Water Intervals, (4) The Deep Waterpower Workout, (5) The Waterpower Warm-Down, (6) The Waterpower Workout, (7) The Twenty-five-Minute Powerhouse Workout, (8) Gait Training, (9) Specific Rehabilitation Exercises (SREs), (10) Resistance Training, and (11) Sport-Specific or Dance-Specific Workout. Use the chart below to know which exercises to do during each phase of your rehabilitation. (This chart applies to all nonsurgical upper-body injuries except injuries to the neck. Because the exercises for the neck are vastly different from the others, they have been treated separately in their own category. The chart for the neck that guides you through your rehab phases appears on pages 290 and 291.)

Components of a Water Healing Workout for Upper Body, Nonsurgical and Postsurgical

Injuries to: shoulder, elbow, wrist, and hand

Phase 1

1. Shallow-Water Walking Warm-Up (Exercise 24, page 264)
2. Stretching
3. The Waterpower Warm-Down (for severe injury)
   OR The Waterpower Workout, Level 1. For either, use caution with all arm movements.
4. Specific Rehabilitation Exercises (SREs)—braced
   One set of ten reps
5. Stretching
6. **ICE**

Phase 2

1. Shallow-Water Walking Warm-Up (Exercise 24, page 264)
2. Stretching
3. The Waterpower Workout, Level 1. Use caution with all arm movements.
4. SREs—braced, but gradually increasing speed
   Two sets of ten reps
5. Stretching
6. **ICE**

Shoulder

The shoulder is the most mobile and uniquely designed joint in the body. The joint between the scapula (shoulder blade) and the humerus (upper-arm bone) is so unstable it is held together mostly by an extensive system of ligaments, tendons, and muscles. The scapula is a triangular free-floating bone on the back of the rib cage. Only a short ligament holds the scapula to the clavicle (collarbone), which then connects to the central skeleton. This loosely connected arrangement allows for incredible mobility, yet the shoulder girdle, as this entire structure is called, is often asked to generate extreme force.

The most common shoulder injuries are **shoulder separations**—sprains or tears of the ligaments that connect the clavicle to the scapula; **shoulder dislocations**—the joint capsule and intrinsic tendons are stressed to the point that the humerus is actually

The
Complete
Waterpower
Workout
Book

274

Phase 3

1. Shallow-Water Walking Warm-Up (Exercise 24, page 264)
2. Stretching
3. The Waterpower Workout. Progress from Level 2 to Level 3; begin to use arms as normally as possible.
4. Sport-Specific or Dance-Specific Workout (optional)
5. SREs with resistance
   Two sets of twenty reps
6. Stretching
7. **ICE**

Phase 4

1. Shallow-Water Walking Warm-Up (Exercise 24, page 264)
2. Stretching
3. The Twenty-five-Minute Powerhouse Workout
4. Sport-Specific or Dance-Specific Workout (optional)
5. SREs, resistance plus speed
   Three sets of twenty reps
6. Stretching
7. **ICE**

pulled out of the socket; **muscle strains or tears** of the deltoids, biceps, or the muscles of the rotator cuff; or a **broken clavicle**—the collarbone fractures from impact.

An injury to any of the parts of the shoulder's support system reduces the effectiveness of the entire joint. The most important thing you can do to speed the healing of a shoulder injury is to strengthen the muscles that surround the joint, the entire shoulder girdle, and the adjacent joint, the elbow.

For the first few sessions, do the full series of exercises one arm at a time. Use the healthy arm first to learn the movement and the coordination, then slowly repeat the entire series with the injured arm remaining within your pain-free range of motion. By Phase 3, when the inflammation of your injured shoulder is reduced and the muscles gain strength, you can do the exercises with both arms simultaneously, controlling the strong arm so it works at the speed dictated by the healing arm. Through the first three phases of rehabilitation, always keep your arm in the water. This is a built-in safeguard that avoids dangerous overhead movements.

Specific
Rehabilitation
Exercises for
the Upper Body

275

Exercise 1. Dig Deep *See Exercise 28, page 64.*

Exercise 2. Rotator Cuff Swings

Teres minor, teres major, pecs, infraspinatus, subscapularis

Stand in shoulder-deep water by the side of the pool. If your right shoulder is injured, hold the side of the pool with your right hand. Use any bracing position that does not cause pain in the shoulder. Learn the movement with your noninjured arm first, then turn to perform your reps with the injured arm.

Tuck your elbow into your ribs and bend it 90 degrees. Hold your hand straight forward, thumb toward the surface of the water (Photo 2A). Hold your upper arm against your body and working within your pain-free range only sweep your forearm out to the position shown in Photo 2B, then back beyond the starting position. Rotate as far as you can while you keep your elbow tucked to your side.

2A

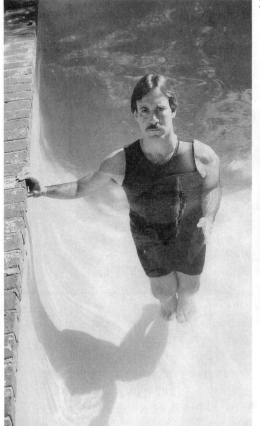

2B

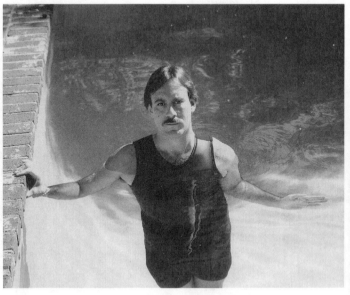

Exercise 3. Front/Back Pull *(Exercise 26, page 62)*

Exercise 4. Up/Down Pull *(Exercise 27, page 63)*

Exercise 5. Lateral Bar Swings
Deltoids, pecs, supraspinatus, teres major and minor, rhomboids

Stand in shoulder-deep water and push an Instructional Swim Bar straight down in front of your hips. Keeping your arms straight, gently swing it from side to side (Photo 5), reaching as far as you can in each direction without aggravating your injury.

5

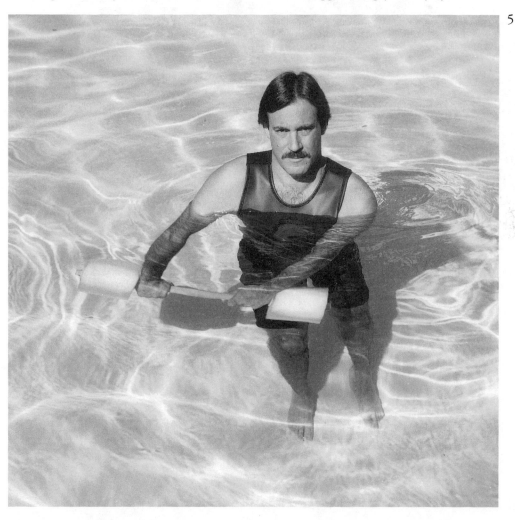

Exercise 6. Cross-Chest Stretch

Posterior deltoids, teres major and minor, infraspinatus, rhomboids, trapezius

Stand in chest-deep water with your weight evenly distributed on both feet, your knees slightly bent so your shoulders are under the water. Grasp the elbow of your healthy shoulder and pull it to the position in Photo 6. Adjust the height of the elbow to avoid pain. Hold as you take three deep, slow breaths. Now *gently* repeat with the injured shoulder.

6

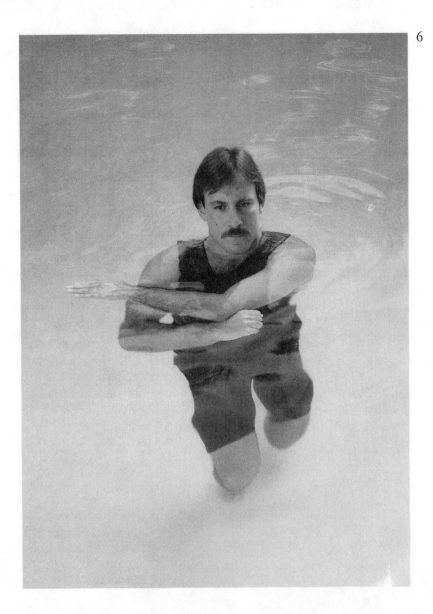

The
Complete
Waterpower
Workout
Book

278

Exercise 7. Overhead Tricep Stretch
Triceps, lats, teres major and minor, infraspinatus

Continue standing in a balanced position with your shoulders under the water and your knees slightly bent. Raise the healthy arm overhead, bending the elbow to touch your fingers to your back between the shoulder blades. Grasp the bent elbow with your other hand and slowly pull, gently increasing the stretch (Photo 7). Hold as you take three slow, deep breaths. Slowly repeat with the affected arm.

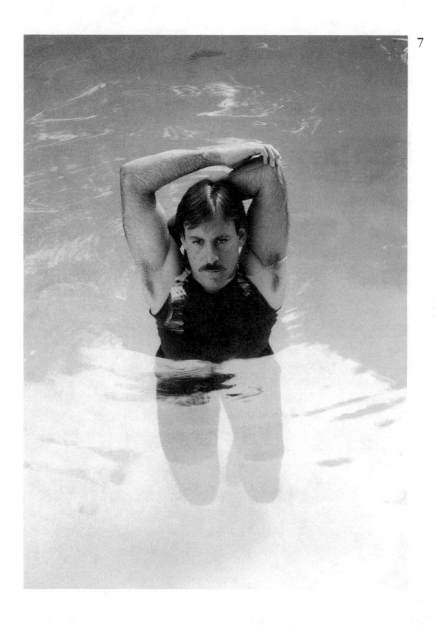

7

Specific
Rehabilitation
Exercises for
the Upper Body

Exercise 8. Penguin Stretch

Infraspinatus, teres minor, deltoids, trapezius, rhomboids

Continue standing in a balanced position with your knees bent and your shoulders under the water. Place your fists on the crest of your pelvis as in Photo 8. Keep your shoulders down as you gently pull both elbows forward. Hold for three slow breaths.

8

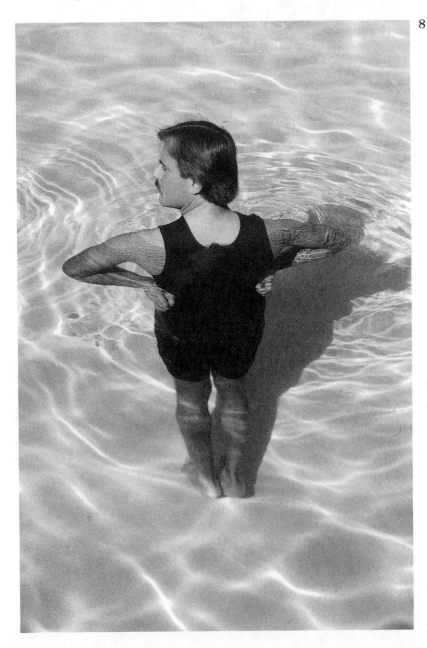

The
Complete
Waterpower
Workout
Book

280

Exercise 9. Bicep Stretch
Biceps, brachialis, deltoids

Stand with your back to the side of the pool or sit on a low step. Reach your straight arm behind you and place it on the deck or a high step, the thumb of your fist down. Slowly lower your body to increase the stretch (Photo 9). Take one slow breath at each increase in stretch.

9

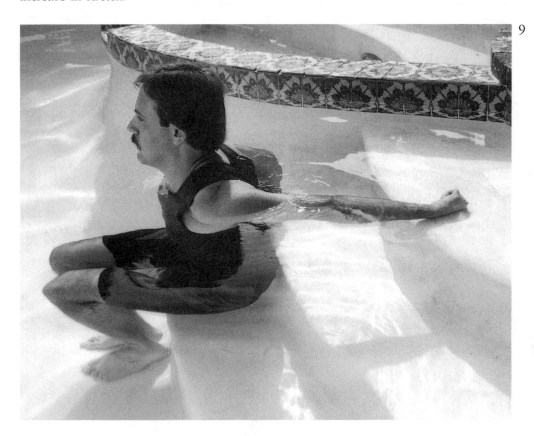

Elbow

The elbow joint is the connection between the upper-arm bone (humerus) and two long bones of the forearm, the radius and the ulna. The lower end of the humerus serves as an anchor location for the many muscles that move the fingers, hand, wrist, forearm, and elbow. With so many muscles attached to such a small spot, the spot is vulnerable to stress and subsequent breakdown. The muscles that clench the fingers into a fist and curl the wrist toward the smooth part of the forearm are located on the inner part of the forearm and attach to the medial epicondyle, commonly called the "funny bone." Inflammation of the tendons that attach to this bone is called **"golfer's elbow."** The muscles on the opposite side of the forearm extend the fingers and wrist to a cocked position and attach to the lateral epicondyle. Inflammation of the tendons that attach here is called **"tennis elbow."** Both of these anchor spots can become inflamed from repetitive stress activities (long hours at the computer, the piano, or at sports) or one-time trauma (an overzealous throw from the outfield to home plate). The large muscles of the upper arm, the biceps, and the triceps also anchor in the elbow region, and can be responsible for pain.

Use these water exercises to strengthen the muscles surrounding the elbow and soothe inflamed tissues nearby. If you have golfer's- or tennis-elbow pain, wear an elbow strap during all of the exercises.

Exercise 10. Arm Curls (Exercise 29, page 65)

The
Complete
Waterpower
Workout
Book

282

Exercise 11. Wrist Curls
Wrist flexors and wrist extensors

Bend your elbows to 90 degrees, and tuck them to your sides. Hold the arms still, wrists cocked back so the palms face forward (Photo 11A). Flex your wrists downward (Photo 11B), then return to the starting position, reaching for maximum range of motion. Perform the sets and reps applicable to your phase. (See chart, pages 274 and 275.)

11A

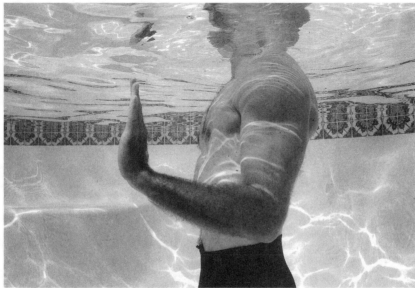

11B

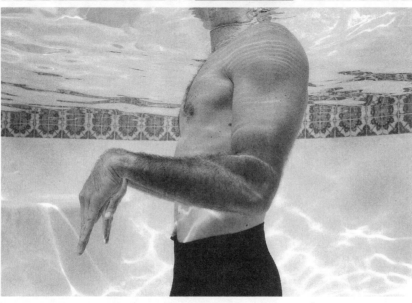

Exercise 12. Hand Rotations
Forearm pronators and wrist supinators

Learn this movement first with your healthy arm. Then apply an elbow strap to the injured arm, bend your elbow and hold your hand in front of you, palm up (Photo 12A). Rotate your hand so the palm faces the bottom of the pool (Photo 12B), then back toward the surface of the water. Complete your required number of sets and reps with your injured arm.

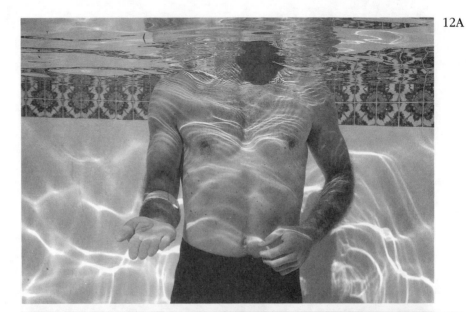

12A

12B

The
Complete
Waterpower
Workout
Book

284

Exercise 13. Wrist Flexor Stretch
Wrist flexors

Try this first with your unaffected arm, then the injured one. Tuck your elbow to your side and bend it to 90 degrees. Grasp the fingers of your affected arm and pull your entire hand to the position in Photo 13A. Then slowly increase the stretch by straightening your elbow to the position shown in Photo 13B. Hold this position as you take three slow breaths. Do this three times, releasing between stretches.

13A

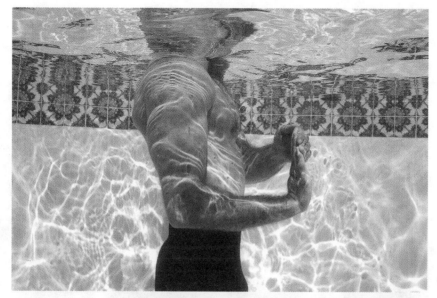

13B

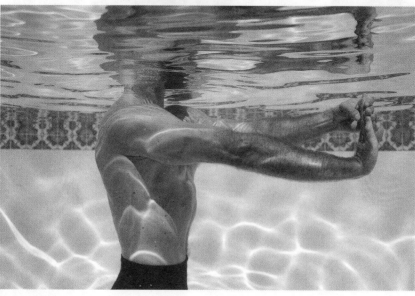

Exercise 14. Wrist Extensor Stretch

Wrist extensors

Do this with the healthy arm first, then the injured one. Tuck your elbow into your side. With your other hand, *gently* push your fingers and hand down as in Photo 14A. Then slowly increase the stretch by straightening your elbow to the position shown in Photo 14B. Hold this position as you take three slow breaths. Do this three times, releasing between stretches.

14A

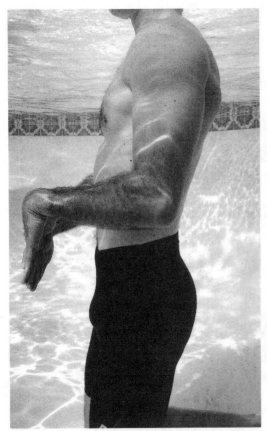

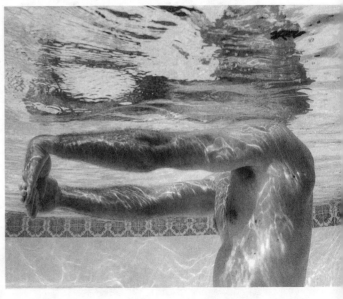

14

The
Complete
Waterpower
Workout
Book

286

Wrist

The small bones of the wrist are arranged in two rows that allow for gliding movement and make many delicate, refined motions possible. These bones are susceptible to fractures due to falls and other trauma. They are slow to heal, and immobility during bone healing creates reduced range of motion and strength. The muscles that move the wrist, hand, and fingers are located in the forearm and, along with the surrounding ligaments, provide strength and stability for the wrist. Common injuries to these tissues are **tendinitis** and **ligament sprains.**

These exercises will help you return to full function of the wrist.

Exercise 15. Wrist Curls *(Exercise 11, page 283)*

Exercise 16. Hand Rotations *(Exercise 12, page 284)*

Exercise 17. Lateral Hand Swings
Radial and ulnar deviators

Hold a SpaBell in your uninjured hand, your arm firmly held against your side. Without moving your shoulder or your elbow, lift your hand so your thumb moves toward the surface of the water (Photo 17A). Then, swing your hand backward so the little finger reaches as far behind you as possible (Photo 17B). Now that you have mastered the coordination, repeat the appropriate number of reps with your injured hand.

17A

17B

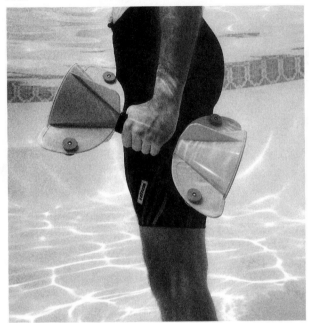
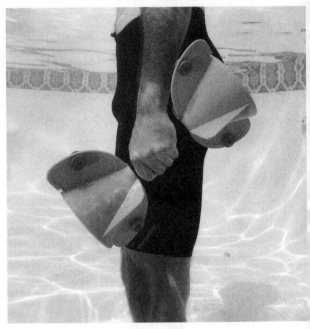

Exercise 18. Wrist Flexor Stretch
(Exercise 13, page 285)

Exercise 19. Wrist Extensor Stretch
(Exercise 14, page 286)

The
Complete
Waterpower
Workout
Book

288

Neck

The neck is the uppermost portion of the spinal column and is made up of the seven cervical vertebrae. Because the neck has more mobility than any other part of the spine, it requires a greater muscular support system. These muscles are vulnerable to strain, because the neck is the area of the body most prone to postural stress. For example, a secretary's neck is strained cradling the telephone between his or her ear and shoulder all day long; a computer operator twists his or her neck looking at copy that is not well placed; the sports fan spends long hours on the sofa watching TV with his or her head tilted on an overstuffed pillow. Although these common daily activities may seem pain free at the time you do them, any aberrant position of the head and neck that is held for very long can lead to strain and resulting pain that occurs hours later or even the next day. The muscles of the neck are a common source of shoulder, neck, or headache pain. Poor posture leads to adaptive shortening of the muscles and connective tissue surrounding the neck. Poor posture also places abnormal stress on the cervical vertebrae, which in turn can result in **joint problems like arthritis,** and **disk injury.** Muscular imbalances in the upper back often lead to postural deviations.

Arthritic changes can also be the long-term result of trauma such as whiplash or falls. Although cervical disks can bulge or become herniated, they are less likely to do so than the lumbar disks.

Neck injuries, pain, and discomfort are treated similarly to back problems. Postural problems are corrected by stretching tight muscles and connective tissue and strengthening weakened muscles in the neck, upper back, and chest.

Icing the neck and upper-back muscles is crucial to breaking the strain/pain/muscle spasm cycle common to all neck injuries. Icing often eliminates neck and headache pain immediately. Try it!

Jumping exercises would probably aggravate your neck, so your workout consists mostly of shallow-water walking and The Deep Waterpower Workout. Except when doing your specific rehab exercises, focus on holding your head and neck in a level, neutral position—neither up nor down, turned neither to the left nor to the right. Be sure you have adequate flotation in your deep exercises. If your flotation device doesn't hold you high enough in the water, you will have a tendency to lift your chin and thus extend your neck, possibly causing strain. If The Deep Waterpower Workout exercises increase your pain, try the assisted-swimming exercises in the Back section of Chapter 9. First, perform Exercise 16 (page 255), then assisted-swimming exercises 17 through 21 (pages 256 to 260). Place a second flotation belt under your neck for a pillow during exercises 19, 20, and 21.

If even these gentle exercises cause pain, take the weight of your head completely off your neck by going *under* the water for your exercise program as shown in Exercises 20 through 27, below. Exercises 20 through 23 stretch and strengthen the neck muscles to improve their function and reduce pain. Exercise 27 helps you increase the strength in your upper back to improve daily posture and eliminate future pain. See page 254 for tips on creating a tight seal with your face mask. **As you first learn these exercises, ask your training partner or therapist to grasp the tip of the snorkel lightly so it won't go under the water causing you to choke or make a sudden movement.**

Components of a Water Healing Workout for the Nonsurgical Neck

Phase 1

1. Shallow-Water Walking Warm-Up (Exercise 24, page 264)
2. Specific Rehabilitation Exercises (SREs, submerged)
   One set of three reps, exercises 20 through 23
   Learn exercises 24 and 25, then for Exercise 26, Intervals,
   use Level 1 from Deep Waterpower, (Exercise 3, page 92)
   Do not do Exercise 27 until Phase 3.
3. **ICE.**

Phase 2

1. Shallow-Water Walking Warm-Up (Exercise 24, page 264)
2. SREs (submerged)
   One set of five reps, exercises 20 through 23
   Level 2 Deep Waterpower Intervals (Exercise 8, page 98)
   Do not do Exercise 27 until phase 3.
3. Deep Waterpower Exercises, Level 1 (no intervals, no abdominal exercises if
   they strain the neck)
5. **ICE**

The
Complete
Waterpower
Workout
Book

290

Phase 3

1. Deep-Water Running and Walking Warm-Up
2. Deep Waterpower, Level 1, including Intervals with head above water
3. Sport-Specific and Dance-Specific Work (optional)
4. SREs—exercises 20 through 23 and 27 (page 299)

   Two sets of five reps
5. **ICE**

Phase 4

1. Deep-Water Running and Walking Warm-Up
2. SREs—Exercises 20 through 23, two sets of five reps,

   Exercise 27 do two sets of ten reps
3. The Deep Waterpower Workout, Level 2, progressing to Level 3, OR The Waterpower Warm-Down at beginning of phase, gradually progressing to Waterpower, then The Twenty-Five-Minute Powerhouse Workout
4. **ICE**

Exercise 20. Submerged Neck Flexion
Erector spinae, trapezius, sternocleidomastoids, scalenes

Seal your face mask in place and breathe through your snorkel. Lean back against the side of the pool with your knees bent to keep your head just below the surface of the water. Ask your therapist or training partner to make sure your snorkel stays out of the water. Lower your chin toward your chest (Photo 20), then lift it back to the starting position. Move slowly and carefully. Repeat several times, breathing slowly.

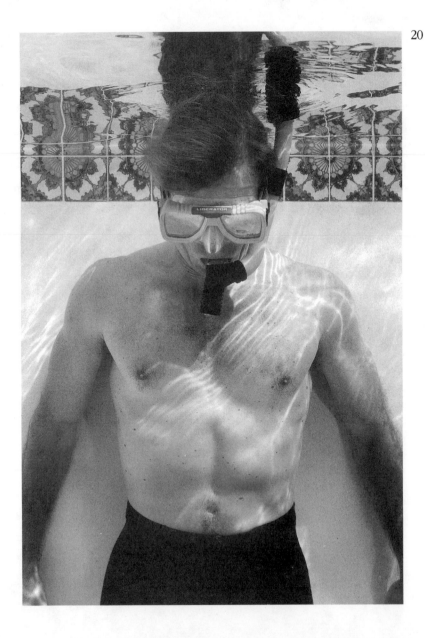

20

The
Complete
Waterpower
Workout
Book

292

Exercise 21. Submerged Neck Rotations

Sternocleidomastoids, trapezius, erector spinae, splenius

Remain in your braced position at the wall, face mask in place, breathing through your snorkel. Hold your shoulders still, keeping them relaxed and down. Slowly turn your head to the left (Photo 21), trying to place your nose directly over your left shoulder. Repeat to the right, then twice more in each direction.

21

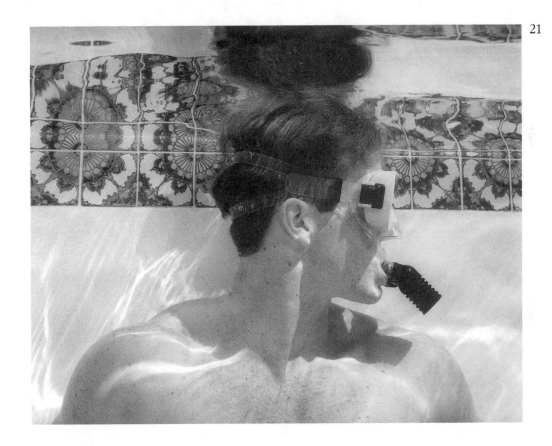

Exercise 22. Submerged Neck Tilt

Splenius, erector spinae, trapezius, sternocleidomastoids, scalenes

Remain braced at the side of the pool, breathing through your snorkel. Keep your nose pointing straight forward as you lean your head to the left, aiming your ear toward your left shoulder (Photo 22). Slowly lift your head back to neutral, then lower it to the right. Breathe slowly and deeply as you do this slowly several times, alternating sides.

22

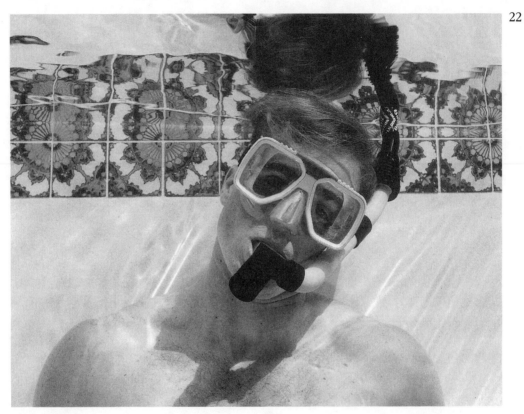

The
Complete
Waterpower
Workout
Book

294

Exercise 23. Submerged, Partial Neck Circles

Trapezius, sternocleidomastoids, scalenes, splenius, levator scapulae

Remain braced at the side of the pool, breathing through your snorkel. Your therapist or training partner will hold the snorkel to make sure it doesn't drop below the surface of the water. Drop your chin forward, then roll your head to the right, reaching your right ear to your right shoulder. Stop there, then let your head roll forward so your chin is down again. Swing your head left, reaching your left ear toward your left shoulder. Roll your head back and forth several times as you breathe slowly.

Because the human body has a specific gravity near that of water, we generally float just below the surface of the water. Exactly where you float depends on whether your lungs are empty or full of air and whether you have a high or low percentage of body fat. If your body-fat percentage is extremely high, you will tend to float, making it necessary to add a weight belt for exercises 24 through 26. Scuba-diving shops can give you weight belts and weights in one- or two-pound increments. If your body-fat percentage is extremely low, you will tend to sink, requiring the addition of some flotation. J&B Foam (see Appendix) makes a one-, two-, or three-square modular flotation belt. **Always have an observer or training partner with you, and remain tethered through the underwater exercises for safety.** Even if you have the pool entirely to yourself, you will probably become disoriented after several minutes under water. In a public pool, take a training partner or friend with you to time your intervals as well as protect your space. Otherwise others in the pool will be unlikely to see you and may swim on top of you.

Exercise 24. Submerged Water Running

Pecs, deltoids, biceps, lats, rhomboids, trapezius, hip flexors, hip adductors,
gluteus maximus, hamstrings, quads

Tether yourself to the side of the pool. Seal your face mask in place. Breathe through your snorkel and slowly begin water running as in Exercise 1 on page 88. Without a flotation device, you will slowly sink below the water (Photo 24). Run like this until you become accustomed to the new sensation, at least two to three minutes. If you feel neck strain, slow your pace.

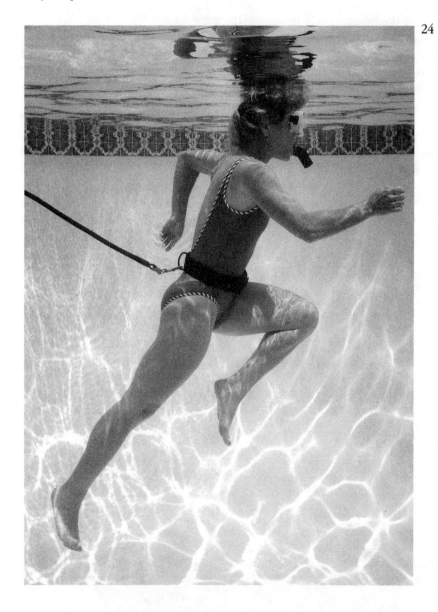

24

The
Complete
Waterpower
Workout
Book

296

Exercise 25. Submerged Water Walking

Hip flexors, gluteus maximus, deltoids, lats, pecs, hamstrings, quads, hip adductors, trapezius, rhomboids, triceps

Remain in the same tethered, underwater position as you straighten your arms and legs to begin water walking (Photo 25). Once again, start slowly until you become accustomed to this new sensation. Walk slowly two to three minutes. If you feel neck strain, slow your pace. (See Exercise 2, page 90, for correct form and variations.)

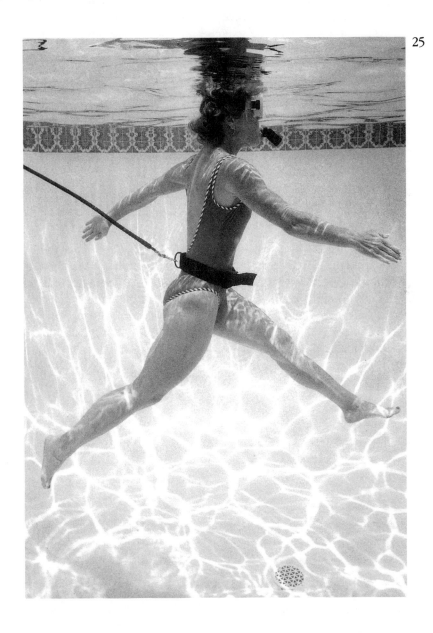

25

Exercise 26. Submerged Intervals
See exercises 24 and 25 for muscle groups.

Your coach, therapist, or training partner can clock your intervals for you by whistling at the beginning and end of each interval, or you can count arm strokes instead of counting seconds. Count "one" every time your right hand comes forward. Start with the intervals in Level 1 on page 92.

Exercise 27 appears in your exercise charts only in phases 3 and 4 of rehabilitation. It requires more direct muscular involvement of the upper back and other postural muscles. Consider it a maintenance exercise after you have gone through the acute phases of rehab.

Exercise 27. One-Way Arm V Lifts
Posterior deltoid, rhomboids, trapezius, erector spinae, infraspinatus, teres minor, triceps, anterior deltoid

Remove your face mask and snorkel. Stand in shoulder-deep water, then bend your knees so your shoulders are under the water. Straighten both arms in front of your hips with your hands angled toward each other (Photo 27A). Lift both arms up and back as far as you can comfortably reach (Photo 27B), then turn the hands to slice through the water with little resistance for a return to the starting position. By working this exercise only one way, you correct the muscle imbalance that causes round shoulderedness and for many people leads to neck pain.

**The
Complete
Waterpower
Workout
Book**

298

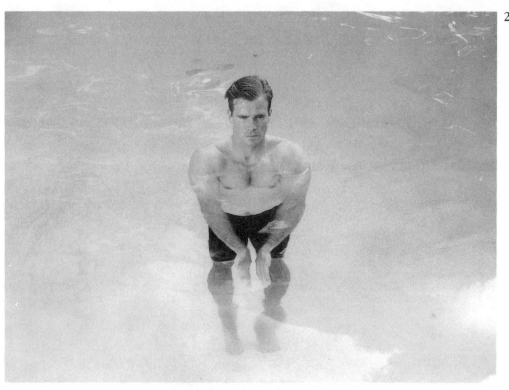

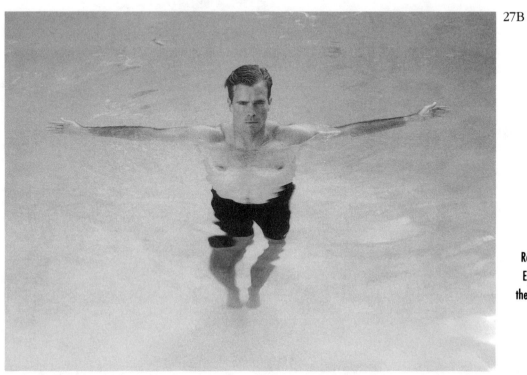

Specific
Rehabilitation
Exercises for
the Upper Body

Specific Rehab Exercises—Upper Body

See chart on pages 274 and 275 for numbers of sets and reps.

See chart on pages 274 and 275 for numbers of sets and reps.

Shoulder

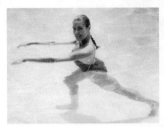 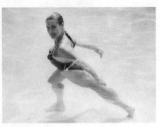

1. Dig Deep

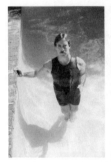 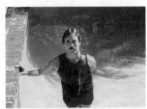

2. Rotator Cuff Swings

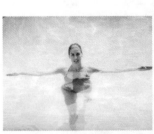 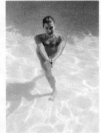

3. Front/Back Pull

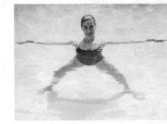 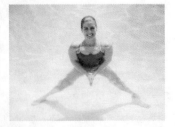

4. Up/Down Pull

The
Complete
Waterpower
Workout
Book

300

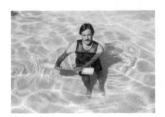

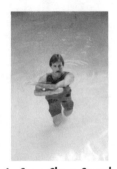

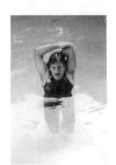

5. Lateral Bar Swings

6. Cross-Chest Stretch
One to two reps each side

7. Overhead Tricep Stretch
One to two reps each side

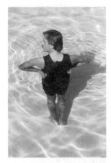

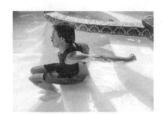

8. Penguin Stretch
One to two reps each side

9. Biceps Stretch
One to two reps each side

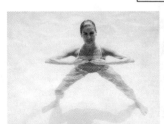

Elbow

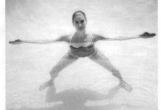

10. Arm Curls

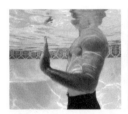

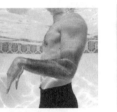

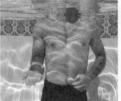

11. Wrist Curls

12. Hand Rotations

Specific
Rehabilitation
Exercises for
the Upper Body

301

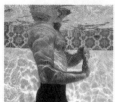
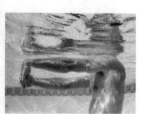
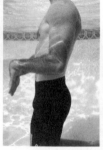

13. Wrist Flexor Stretch
One to two reps each side

14. Wrist Extensor Stretch
One to two reps each side

Wrist

15. Wrist Curls
16. Hand Rotations

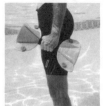
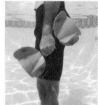

18. Wrist Flexor Stretch
One to two reps each side

19. Wrist Extensor Stretch
One to two reps each side

17. Lateral Hand Swings

Neck

See chart on pages 290 and 291 for numbers of sets and reps

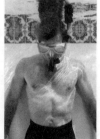
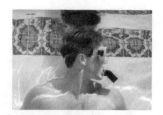
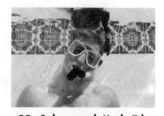

20. Submerged Neck Flexion   21. Submerged Neck Rotation   22. Submerged Neck Tilt

23. Submerged Partial Neck Circles

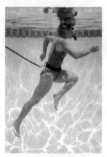
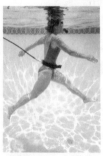
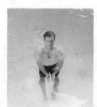
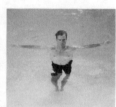

The
Complete
Waterpower
Workout
Book

302

24. Submerged
Water Running

25. Submerged
Water Walking

26. Submerged
Intervals

27. One-Way Arm V Lifts

Postsurgical Water Healing

Written with orthopedic surgeon Dan Silver, M.D.

I njured athletes, dancers, and other active people would like nothing better than to go to their local doctor, take a magic one-day pill or treatment for whatever ails them, and go right back to their sport or dance without missing a beat. But when surgery is required, tissues must have time to heal, and the different kinds of tissues heal at varying rates. In some cases the healing takes several days; but for bones to knit, tendons to mend, and muscle, skin, and connective tissue to heal, several weeks are often necessary.

In recent years, orthopedic surgeons have learned new techniques that are less invasive to the body. They now make only small incisions or punctures to insert tiny viewing instruments and microsurgical tools to perform what are called arthroscopic (inside the joint) surgeries. Dr. Dan Silver was one of the first to place a camera on the end of a fiber-optic tube, sending its picture to a TV monitor so surgeons could see inside the body. In this way they can remove, repair, and replace damaged cartilage, tendons, and even fragments of bone without the long incisions that formerly took weeks or even months to heal. The smaller the incision, the less the damage to the body, and the shorter the recovery or downtime.

A change in postsurgical therapy has also helped shorten recovery time. For example, in the past, casts were often worn after knee ligament surgery for eight to twelve weeks, resulting in secondary damage to the joint and surrounding tissues—atrophy (muscle loss), stiffness, and scar tissue. Today, modern orthopedists advocate moving the joint immediately after surgery. They use machines such as the CPM (continuous passive motion) machine to give guided motion during sleep or when the patient is reading or watching television. This continuous motion lubricates the joint, keeps the muscles moving, and prevents the adhesions (scarring) within a joint that cause later stiffness and limited motion. Early movement in water helps achieve these same goals.

Water Healing Workouts fit perfectly into your well-designed postsurgical therapy program, because water provides you the safest place for protected, gradual, and guided motion that does not overly stress the joint or site of your repair. You can start Water Healing Workouts early in the postoperative recovery phase, often before other land-based therapy programs would be possible.

It is essential to consult with your surgeon before beginning a postsurgical water healing program. Water therapy can be extremely beneficial, but if exercises are performed incorrectly or too early, there is a risk of delayed healing or even undoing your surgeon's work.

Advantages of Postoperative Water Therapy

Pain reduction. Water tends to decrease the sensation of pain. Therefore you will be more willing to move earlier in your recovery and will discover more movement and function in water than on land.

Less chance of damage to the surgical repair. Because water's buoyancy virtually eliminates gravity, you and your surgeon can be more confident that the repaired tendons or fixed fractures are not going to pull apart during an exercise session.

Quicker return to activity. You no longer have to wait until you can perform weight-bearing moves on land to return to activity. Soon after surgery, your surgeon can feel secure in directing you to water workouts that will help speed you back into activity.

Safer, more efficient workouts. Water exercise provides an accommodating environment of variable resistance. When you are weakened immediately after surgery, and when movement causes pain, you can push easily against the water, encountering little resistance. When you become stronger and more confident, you can push harder against the water and instantly create more resistance. When *you* control the resistance, your therapy program is safer. Thus water is a safer medium than weight-training machines that can be loaded too heavily, causing pain and tissue damage.

The
Complete
Waterpower
Workout
Book

304

After Surgery

When you wake up in the recovery room, you likely feel groggy and your mouth is dry. When you finally remember where you are, you probably focus your attention on the injury that brought you to the operating room in the first place. All you can feel is a bulky, protective dressing around your arm, leg, or on your back. Although you shouldn't make many movements at the surgical site, you keep testing. It feels as if it will take forever to move normally again. This is a natural part of postsurgical recovery. The tissues take time to heal.

For several days or more, bandages prevent the opening in your skin from becoming infected. While you are bandaged, you may be put in a brace or splint specifically designed for your affected body part. Such protective devices keep you from performing any undesirable movement that could harm your surgical site. On the other hand, you may find yourself attached to a machine that moves your postsurgical joint through safe, guided motion during this early recovery time. Only rarely will anyone enter the water during the bandaged stage. The exception is the highly motivated athlete or dancer who requests and receives a fiberglass cast, a waterproof lining, and the approval of the surgeon to begin gentle conditioning exercises while the cast protects the surgical area. Normally, you will wait until the bandages are removed before entering the water. Now your Postsurgical Water Healing Workouts can begin.

Four Phases of Postsurgical Rehabilitation

The four phases of postsurgical rehabilitation closely parallel the four phases of nonsurgical rehab, because the goals are the same: to reduce pain, swelling, and inflammation while increasing range of motion, strength, and function. At the same time, you want to preserve as much fitness as possible. But surgery invades the body's own repair systems by cutting through blood and lymph vessels, nerve fibers, muscles, tendons, and skin. Consequently, as the body tries to reduce swelling and inflammation following surgery, it isn't as effective, because the systems that remove excess fluids and chemicals have been debilitated. Strength is more difficult to regain when the muscles or corresponding tendons have been cut. Flexibility, too, can be dramatically reduced, because your range of motion is limited by increased swelling, the postsurgical scar, and adhesions in the surrounding tissues. After surgery, you will have to work with greater pain, swelling, and stiffness in your movement than in nonsurgical rehab. Each phase in your rehabilitation will be longer in duration with a slightly different emphasis. And you must observe precautions specific to your surgery.

While wound healing is not an issue in nonsurgical rehabilitation, it is the primary consideration in postsurgical rehab. The tiny arthroscopic punctures usually heal in five days, while the larger incisions can take up to two weeks. When your wounds have healed sufficiently for safe immersion in water, you can start to do slow, controlled stretches and movements in water that increase your range of motion and strength.

Wait until your surgeon has inspected the wound to be certain there is no gap or infection. Then you can enter the water. Until recently, most surgeons felt that stitches had to be removed prior to beginning a water-therapy program. But now many postoperative patients go into clean, private pools (not public pools or health clubs) with their stitches in place. Only the larger incisions cause concern about separation of the wound as it gets wet. And even with large incisions, you can usually go into the water after two weeks without any risk. General advice on when to enter the water appears under each surgical procedure in this chapter, but it is always best to **consult your doctor.** Some surgeons allow early movement and early immersion in water; others do not.

Look back at the four phases of rehabilitation presented in Chapter 8 (pages 222 through 224). Your four phases of postsurgical rehab are similar. Only special considerations are listed below.

PHASE 1

- Your wound must be healed enough so there is no danger of its pulling apart in the water.

- Prescribed medication and ice will help you fight pain. Pain inhibits muscle function and slows your recovery by causing increased weakness and stiffness. Eliminating pain speeds recovery, so take your prescribed pain killers and ice the postsurgical site.

- Phase 1 will last longer for you than for someone with a similar injury who did not have surgery, because you will experience more pain, swelling, and inflammation.

- You will need to spend concentrated time on improving your flexibility.

PHASE 2

- Continue aggressive treatment for pain and swelling by icing, bracing, and taking prescribed medications.

- You may have to work *around* some pain, swelling, and inflammation as you try to improve your flexibility, strength, and function, but do not work *through* pain. That is, you can expect to feel some moderate pain when you move the surgical site, but don't force an exercise and increase your pain beyond that moderate level.

- Don't challenge internal surgical repairs during your strength exercises. Strength exercises must be controlled in speed and range of motion to protect bones, tendons, ligaments, and muscles that are being held together by sutures, staples, screws, plates, or pins.

The
Complete
Waterpower
Workout
Book

306

┌─────────────┐
│   PHASE 3   │
└─────────────┘

- You will probably still have decreased flexibility. Nevertheless, you must begin to progress in your aerobic and anaerobic fitness *safely* within the limitations of your range of motion.
- Midway through Phase 3, you will be able to take much of your attention away from protecting the surgical site and begin focusing on regaining full function.
- Now your postsurgical rehab is exactly the same as the nonsurgical Phase 3, Chapter 8 (page 223).

┌─────────────┐
│   PHASE 4   │
└─────────────┘

- Your symptoms are gone, but you aren't yet fit enough to return to full land activity. You must work your way up to 95 percent strength, flexibility, and function before returning to your usual activity.
- Now your postsurgical rehab is the same as the nonsurgical Phase 4 (page 224).

When you have surgery performed on your lower body, you may spend weeks or even months without weight bearing. Therefore, your Water Healing Workout will begin in deep water. The charts on pages 274 to 275, 308 to 310, and 336 to 337 list the components of your Water Healing Workouts by phases. Your Phase 1 workout is simple, brief, and designed to improve your range of motion while keeping you off your feet. You will gradually progress to increased intensity as the wound heals, and to increased weight bearing as you can tolerate it.

Upper-body surgeries allow you to walk normally, so you won't require suspension. You will start in shallow water, but you must take care to protect the postsurgical site. The chart on pages 274 and 275 shows your initial Water Healing Workout and workouts for the succeeding phases.

Because exercises for the neck are vastly different from upper-body and lower-body exercises, they have been treated separately at the end of this chapter. (See chart, pages 336 and 337).

The exercises in this chapter represent the gentlest range of motion and stretching exercises for your postsurgical rehabilitation. They become increasingly more difficult, so do them in the order presented. Let the chart guide you from these gentle exercises to a more forceful, powerful workout as you work your way through Phase 4.

As in all Water Healing Workouts, **begin slowly, move gently, and proceed with caution. If you feel pain, narrow your range of motion or move even more slowly.**

Postsurgical
Water Healing

Components of a Postsurgical Water Healing Workout for Lower Body (Minor Surgery)

Ankle—arthroscopy for removal of loose bodies
Knee—arthroscopy for patellar shaving or meniscus removal
Hip—arthroscopy for removal of torn labrum or loose bodies
Back—microsurgery for laminectomy or diskectomy

Phase 1

1. Deep-Water Running and Walking Warm-Up
2. Stretching
3. The Deep Waterpower Workout, Level 1 (no intervals)
4. Gait Training, wearing flotation device (exercises 24 and 25 only, pages 264 and 265)
5. Specific Rehabilitation Exercises (SREs),
   One set of ten reps
6. Stretching
7. **Ice immediately upon leaving the pool**

Phase 2

1. Deep-Water Running and Walking Warm-Up
2. Stretching
3. The Deep Waterpower Workout, including intervals, Level 2
4. Gait Training, no flotation belt (exercises 24 and 25 only, pages 264 and 265)
5. SREs, gradually increasing speed as tolerated,
   Two sets of ten reps
6. Stretching
7. **ICE**

Phase 3

1. Deep-Water Running and Walking Warm-Up
2. Stretching
3. Deep-Water Intervals
4. Gait Training, no flotation belt (exercises 24, 25, and 26, pages 264 through 266)

The
Complete
Waterpower
Workout
Book

308

5. The Waterpower Warm-Down at start of Phase 3; The Waterpower Workout, Level 2 (no intervals), at end of phase
6. Sport-Specific or Dance-Specific Workout (optional)
7. SREs, slow down and add resistance equipment,
   Two sets of fifteen reps
8. Stretching
9. **ICE**

Phase 4

1. Deep-Water Running and Walking Warm-Up
2. Stretching
3. The Waterpower Workout, Level 2, at start of phase (including intervals); progress to Level 3, then to The Twenty-five-Minute Powerhouse Workout at end of phase
4. Sport-Specific or Dance-Specific Workout (optional)
5. SREs, using resistance equipment and adding speed,
   Two sets of twenty reps
6. Stretching
7. **ICE**

Components of a Postsurgical Water Healing Workout for Lower Body (Major Surgery)

Foot—bunionectomy, displaced fractures
Ankle—tendon transfer, displaced fractures
Knee—lateral release, anterior cruciate ligament repair, posterior cruciate ligament repair, medial collateral ligament repair, lateral collateral ligament repair, internal fixation of fractures, tibial osteotomy
Hip—total hip replacement, fractures that require internal fixation

Phase 1

1. Deep-Water Running and Walking Warm-Up
2. Stretching
3. SREs, slow, emphasizing range of motion,
   One set of ten reps
4. Stretching
5. **ICE immediately upon leaving the pool**

Phase 2

1. Deep-Water Running and Walking Warm-Up
2. Stretching
3. The Deep Waterpower Workout, Level 1, with intervals
4. Gait Training, wearing a flotation device (exercises 24 and 25 only, pages 264 and 265)
5. SREs, gradually increasing speed as tolerated,
   Two sets of ten reps
6. Stretching
7. **ICE**

Phase 3

1. Deep-Water Running and Walking Warm-Up
2. Stretching
3. The Deep Waterpower Workout with intervals, progress from Level 2 at start of phase to Level 3 at end of phase
4. Gait Training without flotation device (exercises 24, 25, and 26, pages 264 through 266)
5. The Waterpower Warm-Down
6. SREs, slow movement with extra resistance equipment,
   Two sets of fifteen reps
7. Stretching
8. **ICE**

Phase 4

1. Deep-Water Running and Walking Warm-Up
2. Stretching
3. The Waterpower Workout, progressing from Level 1 at start of phase to Level 3, or even The Twenty-five-Minute Powerhouse Workout at end of phase
4. Sport-Specific or Dance-Specific Workout (optional)
5. SREs, use resistance equipment and add speed,
   Two sets of twenty reps
6. Stretching
7. **ICE**

The
Complete
Waterpower
Workout
Book

310

Tips for Postsurgical
Water Healing Workouts

- Consult with your surgeon before you begin.

- **Start with the easiest exercises, which are presented first.** Some pain is to be expected when you move the postsurgical site, but if one of the more difficult exercises causes you more than moderate pain, *don't do it.* Back up, then try the exercise gently again in the next session.

- **Ice after each workout.** Icing can make the difference between recovering from a workout or not. If you ice, you may not be sore, stiff, or have as much pain tomorrow.

- **Don't try to do too much.** If pain or swelling increases after the workout and persists after icing, you worked too hard. If you feel increased swelling or stiffness the next morning, reduce your workout intensity—speed and repetitions.

- **Do *only* the Phase 1 exercise components when you are in Phase 1.** When you move to Phase 2 perform *only* the Phase 2 components, and so on.

- **Your crutches can help you into the pool.** Use them going down the steps if your pool doesn't have double railings there. You'll use them to exit the pool as well. Wear your flotation belt or vest into the pool. If your surgeon has given you instructions to *avoid weight bearing,* don't put the leg that was operated on down on the pool bottom. If you are in the *partial weight-bearing* stage, you can begin touching down when you reach chest-deep water. Use your hands to move along the side of the pool to reach chest-deep water.

- **Highly motivated athletes and dancers normally progress themselves quickly through the phases.** Although discomfort and pain are expected during movement of the postsurgical site, residual joint pain after the workout or an increase in pain or swelling tells you that you are moving too fast. Cut back your water workouts and consult with your surgeon.

- **Any fever, increased redness of the wound, or drainage of fluids from the wound should be discussed with your surgeon,** and you should stop all workouts until you have your doctor's permission to resume.

- **For most rapid progress, perform daily Postsurgical Water Healing Workouts through phases 1 and 2.** If that isn't feasible, do at least three Water Healing Workouts a week during Phase 1 and progress to at least three to five workouts a week during phases 2 through 4.

ANKLE AND FOOT

Minor ankle and foot surgeries. Only small skin incisions are required to perform arthroscopies of the ankle or foot, or to remove a cyst or neuroma (bulbous swelling of an inflamed nerve). Five to seven days are normally spent in the bandaged and wound healing stages. None of these procedures requires fixation of bone or repair of tendons, so only light protection against movement is required.

Major ankle and foot surgeries. Reconstruction of the ankle, tendon transfers, and tendon repairs of the foot are major surgeries. So are bunion removals and fracture repairs that require internal fixation (screws, pins, or staples to hold broken bones together). You will probably find yourself in a cast or a splint for two to three weeks after such surgeries to hold the position of the bones, to protect tendons, and to relieve pain caused by movement.

Some surgeons cast such surgeries for as long as six weeks. But if you ask for a *fiberglass cast with a waterproof lining,* the surgeon may allow you to wear the cast into the pool to begin deep-water exercise as soon as the wound has healed. The cast immobilizes the surgical site while the rest of your body continues to train and stay fit. In fact, neurological messages are sent to the immobilized foot and ankle, helping you maintain muscle tone there.

Ask your doctor what was done surgically so you will understand and respect any contraindications (activities not considered safe) you are given and therefore will not disrupt the fixation of any surgical procedures.

You must immobilize your ankle or foot for different lengths of time, depending on whether yours was minor or major surgery. Tape or splint a foot or ankle during the fitness portion of your Postsurgical Water Healing Workout. Remove the tape or splint to perform your specific rehabilitation exercises (SREs).

Exercise 1. Ankle Flexion and Extension
(Exercise 1, page 240)

Exercise 2. Foot Inversion and Eversion
(Exercise 2, page 241)

The
Complete
Waterpower
Workout
Book

312

Exercise 3. Foot Circles
(Exercise 3, page 242)

Exercise 4. Write with Big Toe
(Exercise 4, page 242)

If you've had toe surgery or surgery for the removal of a bunion or neuroma, save exercise 5 and 6 until Phase 3 or 4 (depending on when you can do them painlessly).

Exercise 5. Toe Raises
(Exercise 5, page 243)

Exercise 6. Negative Toe Raises
(Exercise 6, page 244)

In Phase 3, use a swim fin to add resistance to exercises 1 through 4.

KNEE

Minor knee surgery. The most common knee injuries that require surgery are a torn meniscus (cartilage) or chondromalacia of the patella (kneecap). For correction of these conditions, three small punctures are made to allow the surgeon to insert the arthroscope and use microsurgical instruments to remove or trim the cartilage or a portion of the cartilage or to shave off bony irregularities behind the kneecap. The punctures are often closed with one stitch each and they will heal well even if they become wet before the stitch is removed. Following these procedures, there is no risk of pulling a puncture wound apart, so within three to five days after surgery, it is safe for you to enter the water to begin Water Healing.

After knee surgery, you may be missing 15 to 30 degrees of extension, flexion, or both. In other words, you can't completely bend or straighten your knee. Without being able to lock your knee in a straight position, you will find that it feels unstable when you do sideways straight-leg movements. So be careful and cautious as you perform Exercise 13 below.

Postsurgical
Water Healing

Another common knee surgery is a lateral release, which is performed to correct patellar malalignment problems (which lead to chondromalacia). Recovery time is slower from this surgery because of the large amount of work performed under the skin. Bleeding into the area continues for two to three days after the surgery, so movement is discouraged during that time. After the first days, gentle movement is allowed, but you must wait at least seven days to begin water therapy. A portion of the quadriceps muscles is weakened by this surgery, so focus on regaining quad strength.

Major knee surgery. When you tear an anterior cruciate ligament (ACL), or posterior cruciate ligament (PCL) of the knee, it can now be reconstructed arthroscopically. Surgeons usually harvest tissue from the patient's hamstring or patellar tendon to use as a replacement ligament. Although the puncture wounds to the knee are small, the incision to take tissue from the leg can be several inches long when patellar tendon is used. Water therapy must wait until these wounds are healed. Keep in mind that your new ligament has been stapled or screwed onto the bone. Ask your surgeon about the strength of that fixation and exercise accordingly. You don't want to pull that fixation loose. If you had an ACL repaired, emphasize strengthening your hamstring. If the PCL was repaired, focus on strengthening the quadriceps and gastrocnemius. For best protection in the water wear a rigid, functional brace such as the **Stealth** brace designed by Dr. Silver (See photos 12A and 12B, page 317). The Stealth custom brace has an anatomically-shaped hinge and a pump air-bag system that prevents slippage. This lightweight sports brace is custom made and waterproof, even salt-water-proof, making it ideal for all sports and your Water Healing Workout.

Medial collateral ligaments and lateral collateral ligaments are repaired through a small incision; a suture or a staple reattaches the ligament to the bone. Wound healing usually takes five to seven days before water exercise can begin, and you must **wear a brace when doing lateral hops and lateral leg movements or else avoid them.**

Total knee replacements and other large reconstructive repairs use various forms of internal fixation—screws, pins, plates, or staples. It normally takes seven to ten days before the large incisions of these surgeries heal and you can begin water therapy. If cement was used, light weight-bearing in chest-deep water can begin right away, giving you the chance to learn how to walk with your new knees. (See Gait Training exercises 24 and 25 on pages 264 and 265.) If cement was *not* used, you should begin in deep water, waiting at least six weeks before attempting a gradual transition to shallow-water exercises. Communicate closely with your surgeon and ask an expert in water therapy to supervise your first weeks of Water Healing so that you do not disturb the stability of the knee prosthesis.

Begin your specific rehab exercises (SREs) by strengthening the muscles of the adjacent joints—the hips and the ankles. Exercises 7, 8, and 13 below contract the muscles that cross the knee without requiring that you actually bend the knee. Then add exercises 9 through 12 to your program.

The
Complete
Waterpower
Workout
Book

314

Exercise 7. Standing Leg Swings
(Exercise 15, page 251)

Add a Hydro-Tone boot in Phase 3.

Exercise 8. Toe Raises
(Exercise 5, page 243)

Exercise 9. Quad Extensions
(Exercise 34, page 71)

Push with equal force in both directions of this movement for all knee surgeries except ACL and PCL repairs. If you had an ACL repair, gently let your foot drift forward to the straight position, then forcefully pull your heel back, bending the knee. If you had a PCL repair, forcefully push your foot to the straight position, then gently pull the heel to bend the knee. Keep the knees side by side throughout the exercise.

For all knee surgeries except ACL and PCL repairs add a Hydro-Tone boot in Phase 3.

Exercise 10. Passive Quad/Active Hamstring Curl for ACL Repair

Hamstrings

Don't begin this exercise until your rehab has progressed to Phase 3 and you add resistance.

Buckle a Hydro-Fit buoyancy cuff (see photos 10A and 10B below and page 86) around your ankle. Let your foot float forward to the straight-knee position (Photo 10A), then pull hard to the bent position (Photo 10B). The buoyancy cuff will lift the foot for you, eliminating most quad contraction, yet it provides extra work for your hamstrings as you bend. If you have no buoyancy cuff, repeat Exercise 9.

10A

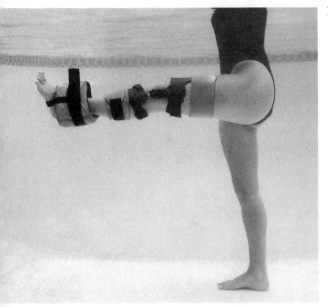

10B

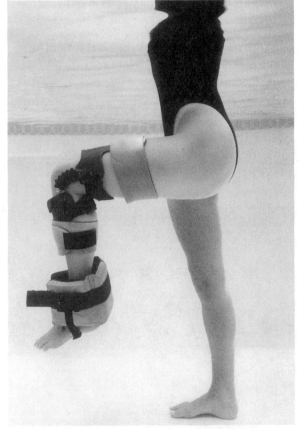

The
Complete
Waterpower
Workout
Book

316

Exercise 11. Hamstring Curls
(Exercise 35, page 72)

Push with equal force in both directions of this movement for all knee surgeries except ACL and PCL repairs. If you had an ACL repair, lift the heel forcefully, but gently return the foot to the pool bottom. If you had a PCL repair, lift the heel gently, then push the foot forcefully to the pool bottom. Keep your knees side by side throughout the exercise.

Exercise 12. Passive Hamstring/Quad Extension for PCL Repair
Quads

Wait until Phase 3 when you add resistance to begin this exercise.

Buckle a Hydro-Fit buoyancy cuff around your ankle. Hold your knees together and slowly let the affected knee bend as the foot floats up to the position in Photo 12A. The buoyancy of the cuff virtually bends your knee for you. Keep your knees together and push your foot down to meet the other foot (Photo 12B). The cuff forces you to work the quads while letting you rest the hamstrings. If you don't have a cuff, repeat Exercise 11. Move your foot **slowly** to the bent position, then work harder as you push your foot to the straight position.

12A
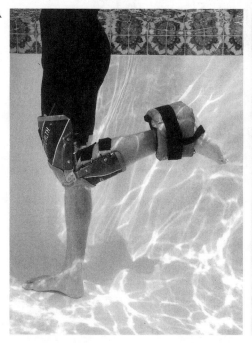

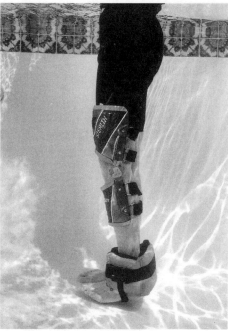
12B

Postsurgical
Water Healing

317

Exercise 13. Lateral Leg Lifts
(Exercise 31, page 67)

Add a Hydro-Tone boot in Phase 3.

Exercise 14. Quad Stretch
(Exercise 36, page 73)

Add this exercise as soon as it becomes possible to do.

Exercise 15. Shallow-Water Walking
(Exercise 24, page 264)

Exercise 16. Marching
(Exercise 25, page 265)

Exercise 17. Front Flutter Kick
(Exercise 23, page 60)

Add fins in Phase 3.

Exercise 18. Back Flutter Kick
(Exercise 18, page 55)

Add fins in Phase 3.

The
Complete
Waterpower
Workout
Book

318

Exercise 19. Floating Squats
Hip flexors, quads, gluteus maximus, hamstrings, hip abductors and adductors

While floating, balance in a squat position with your feet pressed against the sides of an Instructional Swim Bar. (Photo 19A). Slowly stand as the bar sinks lower into the water (Photo 19B), then return to the starting position. In Phase 3, gradually increase power and speed. Stand quickly so your body is half out of the water before you bend your knees and return to the starting position. Then try doing the same exercise on a Water Wafter (Photo 19C). Because this circular piece of equipment has nothing to press your feet against, you must attain a higher degree of balance.

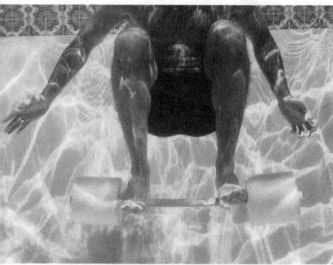

19A

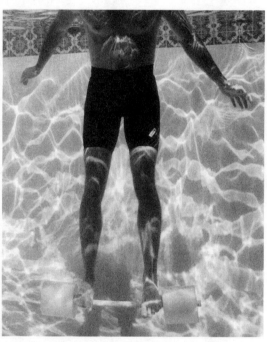

19B

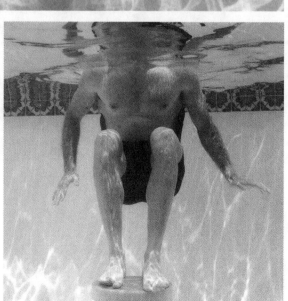

19C

Exercise 20. Tethered Push-Offs

Quads, gluteus maximus, hamstrings, hip adductors, gastroc/soleus complex

Put on your flotation device and tether yourself facing the side of the pool. (For tether information, see page 86). Walk both feet up the side of the pool and gently push off from the side as you lie on your back (Photo 20A). The tether will pull you back to the side of the pool so you can push off again (Photo 20B).

20A

20B

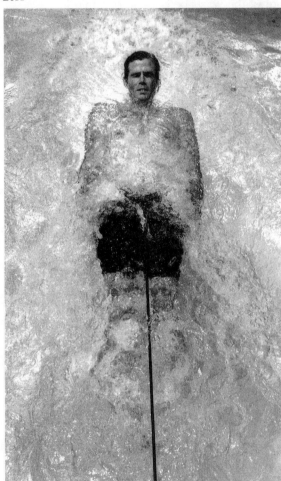
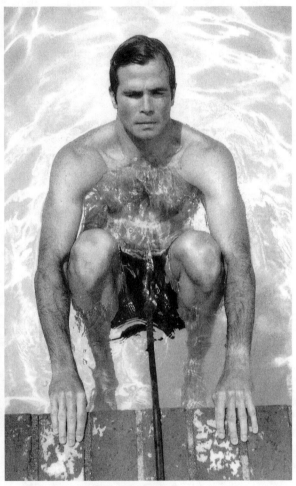

Minor hip surgery. Dr. Dan Silver of Silver Sports Medicine Institute for Arthroscopic Surgery in Century City, California, is one of the pioneers in the use of arthroscopy on the hip for diagnosis and for removing torn labrums (soft-tissue extensions of the hip socket), femoral neck plicae (folds in the lubricating tissue of the joint), and loose bodies (small pieces of free-floating cartilage). After a hip arthroscopy, you will experience three to four days of leakage of saline (surgical cleansing solution) from the puncture wounds. Only after the wounds are completely sealed off and stop leaking can you enter the pool. After that, because there is no concern for disrupting any structures, you can immediately begin your Water Healing Workout.

Major hip surgery. Total hip replacements, the repair of fractures, and hip surgeries that require incisions of four inches or more are considered major hip surgery. Wound healing usually takes seven to ten days. During this time you will probably be allowed to take only short showers, because exposure to water would soften the forming scar. The area around your incision may be painful and ooze tissue fluid for up to two weeks.

Hip-replacement surgeries are often performed in younger adults *without cement,* meaning that the new hip prosthesis is not held in place with bonding materials. Rather, the prosthesis is made of a porous alloy that allows for bone in-growth; in effect, the bone grows into the porous material, making a solid bond. Therefore, you must wait four weeks for that bonding to occur before beginning even suspended water exercise

---

Exercise Precautions
Following Total Hip Replacement

•Do not let your thighbone cross the midline of the body for eight to twelve weeks. Ask your surgeon for specific guidance.

•Avoid hip flexion more than 90 degrees in all total hip surgeries for eight to twelve weeks. Again, ask your surgeon.

•Do not combine hip flexion (bending) with internal rotation (pointing the knee inward).

•Allow four weeks more before beginning water exercise if your surgeon tells you: (1) the femur or pelvis bones are fragile, (2) the trochanter (knob on the top of your femur) was removed and reattached during surgery, or (3) complications during surgery caused a bone fracture.

Postsurgical
Water Healing

and six weeks before starting the gentlest of weight bearing. If *cement* is used to bond your prosthesis in place, you can begin suspended water exercise as soon as the wound heals and you can begin gentle weight bearing four weeks after surgery. Fewer precautions are needed with cement, because the implant is held firmly in place immediately.

Your incision may run vertically up the side of your thigh and buttock, meaning that you can perform early movements in water, because this surgical approach spares crosswise cutting of muscle tissues. However, if your incision runs horizontally from the front to the back of your hip, your surgeons most likely cut directly through the surrounding muscles. Every time you bend your hip, you will be challenging the healing of that incision. Therefore, it will take longer to heal. Before beginning water exercises you must not only wait for the wound to heal, but for the muscles to mend as well.

When a hip fracture has been joined internally by pins or by screws and plates, the surgeon will be able to tell you just how stable the bone is. If you find out that good stability was achieved in surgery, you can enter the water as soon as the wound has healed, usually seven to ten days after surgery.

Add a Hydro-Tone boot during Phase 3 for exercises 21 through 24, and 26.

Exercise 21. Standing Leg Swings
(Exercise 15, page 251)

Exercise 22. Quad Extensions
(Exercise 34, page 71)

Exercise 23. Hamstring Curls
(Exercise 35, page 72)

Exercise 24. Lateral Leg Lifts
(Exercise 31, page 67)

Exercise 25. Knee Swivels
(Exercise 33, page 70)

The
Complete
Waterpower
Workout
Book

322

If you had a hip replacement you should *not* cross the midline of your body with your knee for at least eight to twelve weeks.

Exercise 26. Leg Circles
(Exercise 32, page 68)

Hip replacements: Limit the elevation of your leg to only 45 degrees for the first eight to twelve weeks.

Exercise 27. Flutter Kicking—back, front
(Exercises 18 and 23, pages 55 and 60)

Add fins during Phase 3.

Exercise 28. Combined Stroke—front, back
(Exercises 17 and 19, pages 256 and 258)

BACK

Minor back surgery. Many disk surgeries (laminectomies and diskectomies) today are done arthroscopically or through very small incisions. As with other microscopic surgeries, small punctures are used to minimize damage to the surrounding tissues and cut down the rehabilitation time. Bandages remain in place for five to seven days, then the wound is generally healed. At that time, water therapy can begin even though sutures may still be in place.

Major disk surgery. Complicated laminectomies and surgeries to remove large or multiple disk fragments may require larger incisions. Larger incisions must also be made to perform fusions, or to stabilize a fracture with the use of a rod. Muscle and connective tissue are cut to give the surgeon operating room, and this leads to extended healing time. Bandages are left in place ten days to two weeks. **Get permission from your surgeon to begin Water Healing.**

Exercise 29. Kick, Curl, and Stretch with Flotation Belt, Face Mask, and Snorkel
(Exercise 16, page 255)

Exercise 30. Combined Stroke with Flotation Belt, Face Mask, and Snorkel
(Exercise 17, page, 256)

Exercise 31. Crawl with Face Mask and Flotation Belt
(Exercise 18, page 257)

Wait until Phase 3 to begin this.

Exercise 32. Combined Stroke on Back with Flotation Belt
(Exercise 19, page 258)

Exercise 33. Modified Backstroke with Flotation Belt
(Exercise 20, page 259)

Exercise 34. Backstroke with Flotation Belt
(Exercise 21, page 260)

Wait until Phase 3 to begin this.

The
Complete
Waterpower
Workout
Book

324

Exercise 35. Back Flexion on Bodyciser

Abdominals, hip flexors, quads, erector spinae,
gluteus maximus, hamstrings

Mount the Bodyciser and lie back on it, keeping your arms extended in the water for balance (Photo 35A). Slowly pull the knees and chest toward each other (Photo 35B), then return to the reclining position. If you don't have a Bodyciser, wear your flotation vest or belt and gently perform Exercise 9, Abdominals, from The Deep Waterpower Workout, page 100. Do only the standard version; save the variation until you've progressed to Phase 3.

35A

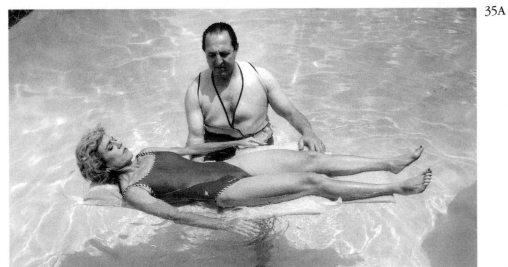

35B

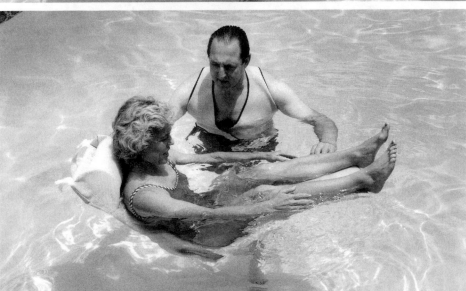

Postsurgical
Water Healing

Ask for your surgeon's approval before attempting exercises 36 and 37.

Exercise 36. Passive Back Extension
(Exercise 22, page 261)

Wait until Phase 3 to begin this.

Exercise 37. Crescent Moon
(Exercise 23, page 262)

Wait until Phase 3 to begin this.

The
Complete
Waterpower
Workout
Book

326

Exercise 38. Knee Twists on Bodyciser
Abdominals, abdominal obliques, quadratus lumborum, sternocleidomastoids

Wait until Phase 3 to begin this. You may wish to have a water exercise expert help you find the exact position the first few times you try it. Starting from the position shown in Photo 35A, page 325, pull your knees to your chest. Slowly twist both knees to the left and turn your head to the right (Photo 38). Now twist both knees to the left and turn your head to the right. If you don't have a Bodyciser, **bend your knees** as you perform Exercise 23, Pendulum, from The Deep Waterpower Workout; page 112.

38

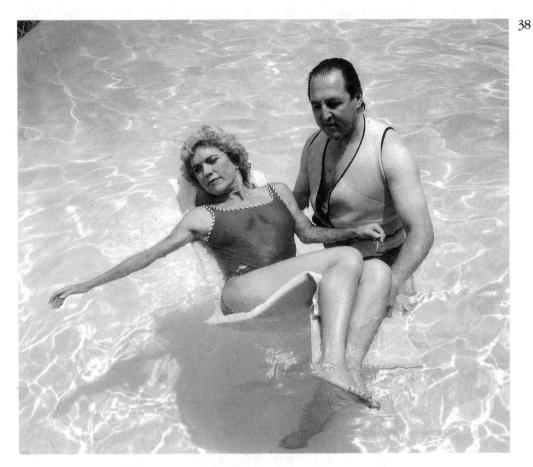

SHOULDER

Minor shoulder surgery. As with other joints of the body, use of the arthroscope generally means little tissue damage occurs and the surgery is considered minor. Today, many small procedures can be performed through the scope: removal of loose bodies (free-floating fragments of cartilage), shaving of irregular bone surfaces, and clipping out of scar tissue. The punctures heal in three to four days and Water Healing can begin.

Major shoulder surgery. The larger, more complicated surgeries of the shoulder include: modified Bankart repair for shoulder, torn labrum and instability repair of the rotator cuff, fixation of fractures, and repair of the acromioclavicular joint (where the collarbone and the scapula meet at the top of your shoulder). Although some surgeons are now repairing rotator cuff tears and labral tears through the arthroscope, the internal work is extensive, and it must still be considered major surgery. Move cautiously not to disrupt any repair where two structures are being held together with internal fixation. Wound healing generally takes seven days, during which time you will most likely wear a sling. Water therapy begins between the second and third week after surgery.

Exercise 39. Arm Curls
(Exercise 29, page 65)

Exercise 40. Dig Deep
(Exercise 28, page 64)

Add Hydro-Tone bells for added resistance on exercises 39 through 41, 43, and 44 when you progress to Phase 3.

The
Complete
Waterpower
Workout
Book

328

Exercise 41. Rotator Cuff Swings
(Exercise 2, page 276)

Exercise 42. Bent-Arm Circles

Deltoids, teres major and minor, infraspinatus, pecs, rhomboids,
supraspinatus, trapezius, biceps

Stand with your knees slightly bent so water covers your shoulders. Bend your arms and touch your fingers to your shoulders with your elbows angled slightly downward. Now draw backward circles with your elbows. Make the circles as large as you can without aggravating the injury, circling only backward. In this way you reinforce good postural alignment.

Exercise 43. Up/Down Pull
(Exercise 27, page 63)

Exercise 44. 30-Degree Arm Lift
Supraspinatus, deltoids, subscapularis, teres major

Stand in neck-deep water with your thumbs touching your thighs. Leading with the little finger, slowly lift your arms to the surface of the water, the arms 30 degrees forward of the lateral plane of the body (Photo 44). Then pull the arm back to the starting position. Learn this movement first with the healthy arm, then perform your reps with the healing arm. Allow the injured shoulder to dictate the speed of both arms.

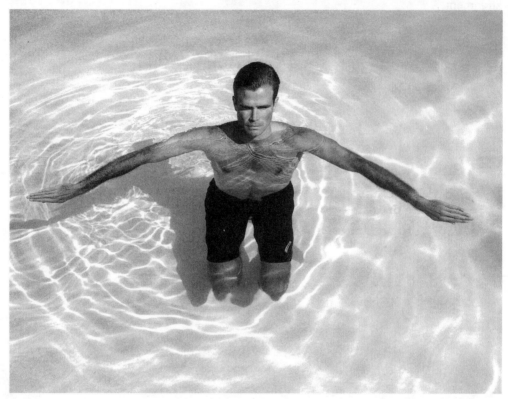

44

The
Complete
Waterpower
Workout
Book

330

Exercise 45. Straight-Arm Circles
Deltoids, pecs, teres major, infraspinatus, trapezius

Extend your arms straight out to the sides just below the surface of the water, palms down. Draw backward circles with your hands. Make the circles as large as you can without causing irritation or pain to the injury. Again, circle only backward to reinforce good posture.

$$\boxed{\text{ELBOW}}$$

Minor elbow surgery. Any surgery to the elbow that requires only two or three punctures is considered minor. Arthroscopies can clear out loose bodies, shave away irregularities of the bone, or clip out scar tissue. Bandages come off after three to five days, at which time you can enter the pool.

Major elbow surgery. When broken bones are held together or tendons attached to bones with screws, staples, or pins, it is considered major surgery. Close communication with your doctor will help you understand the degree of stability of your surgical repair site. It is essential not to disrupt the fixation. Bandages are left in place for seven days, but your water therapy cannot begin until two weeks after surgery. **Consult your surgeon before entering the water and before progressing from one phase to the next.**

Exercise 46. Arm Curls
(Exercise 29, page 65)

Add Speedo SwimMitts for exercises 46 through 48 during Phase 3.

Exercise 47. Wrist Curls
(Exercise 11, page 283)

Exercise 48. Hand Rotations
(Exercise 12, page 284)

Postsurgical
Water Healing

Exercise 49. Lateral Hand Swings
(Exercise 17, page 288)

Do not add the SpaBell until Phase 3.

WRIST AND HAND

Carpal tunnel surgery cuts the ligament across the palm side of the wrist alleviating pressure on the nerves, tendons, and blood vessels that cross into the hand. This surgery can be performed either arthroscopically or through a small incision, which should heal within five to ten days. When fractures of the hand and wrist are severe, they require surgical intervention to reposition and stabilize the bones. Tendons, too, can require surgery for reattachment.

Fractures and tendon repairs require extended immobilization to let the bones and tendons heal in their proper position, which usually means the application of a cast. Rather than become sedentary, ask for a fiberglass cast with waterproof lining so you can continue your water training and not lose fitness while the tissues heal. Do Waterpower or Deep Waterpower workouts until your cast comes off, then begin Phase 1 SREs even though several weeks have passed that normally would have moved you into Phase 2 or 3. Progress through the phases according to how you feel. Slow down your progress if you experience swelling or inflammation, and consult your doctor.

Perform every exercise first with the unaffected hand to learn it. Then apply that learning to the injured side.

Exercise 50. Wrist Circles
Wrist flexors, wrist extensors, radial and ulnar deviators

Tuck your elbow to your side with your elbow bent to 90 degrees. Hold your forearm and elbow stationary as you describe clockwise circles with your hand. The movement occurs *only* at the wrist. Do half your sets and reps clockwise and half your sets and reps counterclockwise.

Exercise 51. Wrist Curls
(Exercise 11, page 283)

Add Speedo SwimMitts in Phase 3.

The
Complete
Waterpower
Workout
Book

332

Exercise 52. Arm Curls
(Exercise 29, page 65)

Add Speedo SwimMitts in Phase 3.

Exercise 53. Write with Forefinger
Wrist flexors and extensors, ulnar and radial deviators

Tuck your elbow against your side and bend your elbow to 90 degrees. "Write" your name using your forefinger as the "pen," moving *only* at the wrist. Once you get the idea, slowly begin again with your injured hand. Write the names of your family members, your best friends, or a line from a favorite song or poem. Instead of counting reps (because you can't count and spell at the same time), write for two thirty-second periods in Phase 1, three thirty-second periods in Phase 2, three one-minute periods in Phase 3, and four one-minute periods in Phase 4.

Exercise 54. Hand Rotations
(Exercise 12, page 284)

Grasp a Hydro-Fit hand buoy in each hand for added resistance during Phase 3.

Exercise 55. Lateral Hand Swings
(Exercise 17, page 288)

Do not add the SpaBell until Phase 3.

Exercise 56. Wrist Flexor Stretch
(Exercise 13, page 285).

Exercise 57. Wrist Extensor Stretch
(Exercise 14, page 286)

Exercise 58. Sponge Squeeze
Finger flexors

Grasp a round or oblong sponge in the palm of your hand. Squeeze gently. Relax, then repeat your number of sets and reps.

    Continue with a thicker, denser sponge in Phase 3.

Exercise 59. Arm Swings
Deltoids, pecs, supraspinatus, infraspinatus, finger and
wrist flexors and extensors

Hold both hands in front of you, elbows slightly bent (Photo 59A). Swing your arms to a wide position (Photo 59B), then back to the starting position. Keep your fingers extended as the muscles in your hand contract to stabilize your wrist against the resistance of the water. In phases 1 and 2, keep your fingers open in a wide position. In phases 3 and 4, hold your fingers together for greater resistance.

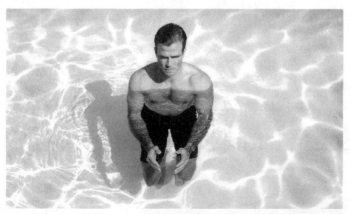

59A

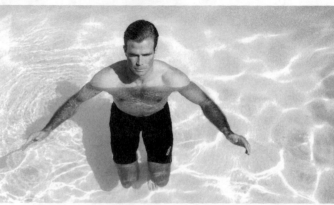

59B

The
Complete
Waterpower
Workout
Book

334

Minor neck surgery. Cosmetic surgery, lymph node biopsies, and the removal of subcutaneous cysts are all minor neck surgeries. Unless muscles had to be cut away during surgery, the only thing that must heal is the skin. In five to seven days, you can enter the water.

Major anterior neck surgery. Cervical disks are removed through small incisions at the front of the neck rather than the back, because access is more direct. When a microscope is used for such diskectomies, the wound will heal in approximately five days. A more complicated surgery from the front of the neck is a fusion, in which a bone block is placed between two vertebral bodies to replace the disk. Although the surgeon stabilizes the bone block, that stability at first is not total, and certain motions in the first six weeks would be dangerous, for they could displace the block. Therefore your surgeon will place you in a rigid cervical collar or brace until an X ray proves that fusion has occurred. Movements of the neck should be no more than 25 degrees in any direction. **Ask your doctor before doing any of these exercises.**

Major posterior neck surgery. Bone spurs can be safely removed from an incision in the back of the neck. The larger the incision, the more muscle soreness you will experience. But because there is nothing to be stabilized, you have less need for caution in movement, and when the wound heals in five to seven days, you can resume whatever range of motion you can perform without pain.

When a posterior cervical fusion is performed, it involves internal fixation, a bone graft, and muscle dissection. The bone graft will take six to ten weeks before it fuses, so you must stabilize your neck in order not to disrupt healing. A rigid cervical collar is worn at all times. After your surgeon views the X ray or CAT scan to verify the bone has grafted, you can enter Phase 1 of your rehabilitation.

Exercises 60 through 63 help you regain mobility and strength in the muscles of your neck. Exercises 64 through 66 offer you fitness exercises that should cause you no neck pain, for you will be submerged and your head will be supported by the water.

Put on a face mask and breathe through the snorkel as you brace yourself with your back pressed against the side of the pool during exercises 60 through 63. (See page 254 for tips on creating a "seal" with your face mask.)

Phase 1

1. Shallow-Water Walking Warm-Up (Exercise 24, page 264)
2. Specific Rehabilitation Exercises (SREs) (submerged)
   Learn exercises 24 and 25 (pages 296 and 297), then for Exercise 26
   (page 298), Intervals, use Level 1 from Deep Waterpower (Exercise 3,
   page 92)
3. **ICE**

Phase 2

1. Shallow-Water Walking
2. SREs (submerged)
   One set of three reps, exercises 20 through 23 (pages 292 to 295)
   Level 2 Deep Waterpower Intervals (page 98)

The
Complete
Waterpower
Workout
Book

336

Exercise 60. Submerged Neck Flexion
(Exercise 20, page 292)

Exercise 61. Submerged Neck Rotations
(Exercise 21, page 293)

Exercise 62. Submerged Neck Tilt
(Exercise 22, page 294)

3. Deep Waterpower Exercises, Level 1 (no intervals, no abdominal exercises if they strain the neck)

4. **ICE**

Phase 3

1. Deep-Water Running and Walking Warm-Up
2. Deep Waterpower, Level 1, including Intervals with head above water
3. Sport-Specific and Dance-Specific Work (optional)
4. SREs—Exercises 20–23 (pages 292 to 295) and 27 (page 298)
   Two sets of three reps
5. **ICE**

Phase 4

1. Deep-Water Running and Walking Warm-Up
2. SREs—Exercises 20–23, two sets of five reps,
   Exercise 27 (page 298), two sets of ten reps
3. The Deep Waterpower Workout, Level 2, progressing to Level 3, OR The Waterpower Warm-Down at beginning of phase, gradually progressing to Waterpower, then The Twenty-five-Minute Powerhouse Workout
4. **ICE**

Exercise 63. Submerged, Partial Neck Circles
(Exercise 23, page 295)

Exercise 64. Submerged Water Running
(Exercise 24, page 296)

Exercise 65. Submerged Water Walking
(Exercise 25, page 297)

Exercise 66. Submerged Intervals

(Exercise 26, page 298)

Exercise 67. One-Way V Arm Lifts

(Exercise 27, page 298)

Do not add this exercise until Phase 3.

The
Complete
Waterpower
Workout
Book

338

Post-Surgical Water Healing Exercise

See chart on pages 308 through 310 for numbers of sets and reps.

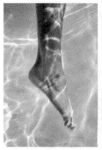 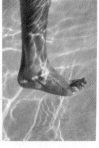

1. Ankle Flexion and Extension

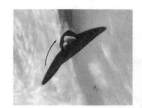 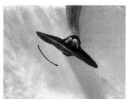

2. Foot Inversion and Eversion

3. Foot Circles
4. Write with Big Toe

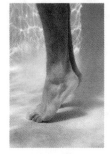 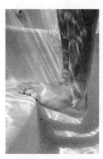

5. Toe Raises

6. Negative Toe Raises

Knee

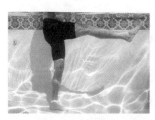 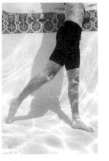 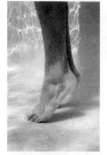

7. Standing Leg Swings

8. Toe Raises

**Postsurgical
Water Healing**

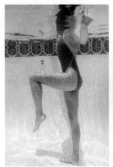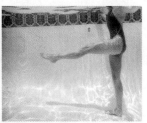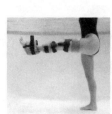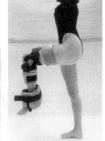

9. Quad Extensions   **10. Quad Extensions for ACL Repair**

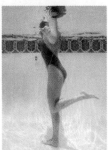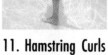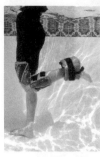

11. Hamstring Curls   **12. Hamstring Curls for PCL Repair**

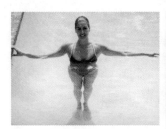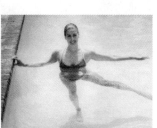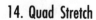

13. Lateral Leg Raises   **14. Quad Stretch**

The
Complete
Waterpower
Workout
Book

340

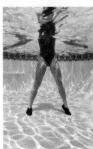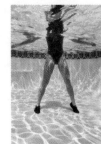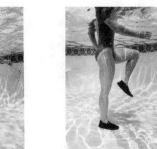

15. Shallow-Water Walking
Forward, backward, sideways

**16. Marching, then marching and lift
on toe**

17. Front Flutter Kick

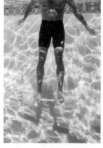

18. Back Flutter Kick

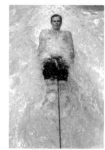
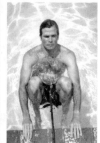

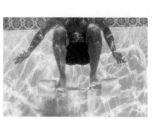

19. Floating Squats

20. Tethered Push-Offs

Hip

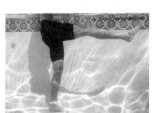
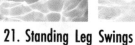
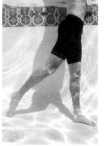
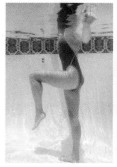

21. Standing Leg Swings

22. Quad Extensions

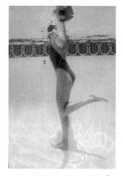
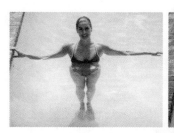

23. Hamstring Curls

24. Lateral Leg Raises

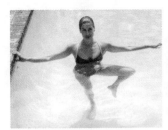
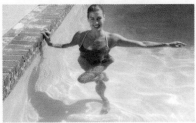

25. Knee Swivels

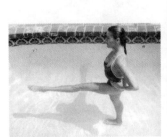
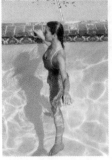
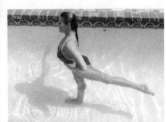

26. Leg Circles

Back

27. Flutter Kicking—front, back

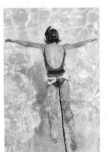
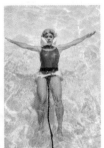

28. Combined Stroke—front, back

The
Complete
Waterpower
Workout
Book

342

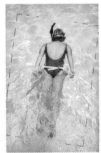
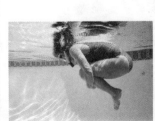
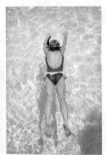

29. Kick, Curl, and Stretch with Flotation Belt, Face Mask, and Snorkel

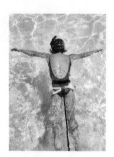

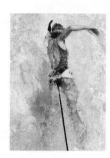

30. Combined Stroke with Flotation Belt, Face Mask, and Snorkel

31. Crawl with Flotation Belt, Face Mask, and Snorkel

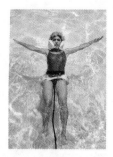

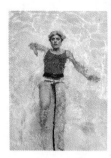

32. Combined Stroke on Back with Flotation Belt

33. Modified Backstroke with Flotation Belt

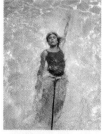

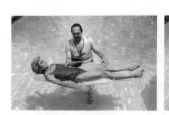

34. Backstroke with Flotation Belt

35. Back Flexion on Bodyciser

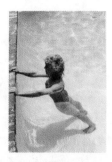

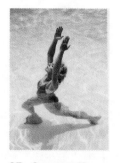

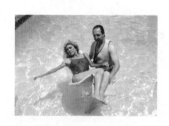

36. Passive Back Extension

37. Crescent Moon

38. Knee Twists on Bodyciser

See chart on pages 274 and 275 for numbers of sets and reps

Shoulder

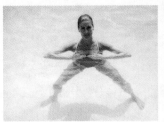 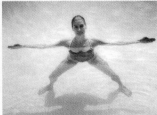

39. Arm Curls

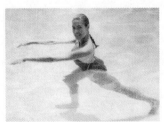 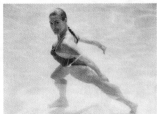

40. Dig Deep

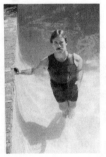

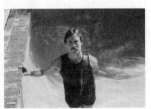

42. Bent-Arm Circles

41. Rotator Cuff Swing

The
Complete
Waterpower
Workout
Book

344

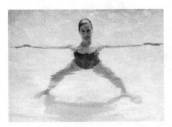 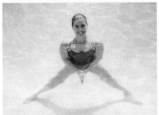

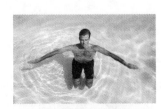

44. Thirty-Degree Arm Lift

43. Up/Down Pull

45. Straight-Arm Circles

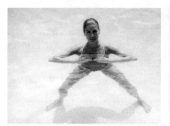
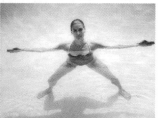

46. Arm Curls

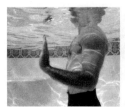
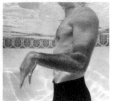

47. Wrist Curls

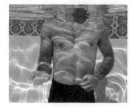
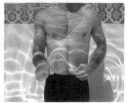

48. Hand Rotations

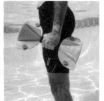
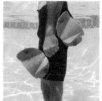

49. Lateral Hand Swings

Wrist and Hand

50. Wrist Circles

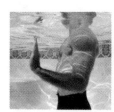
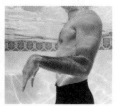

51. Wrist Curls

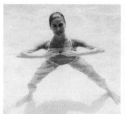
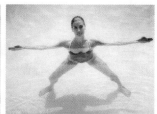

52. Arm Curls

Postsurgical
Water Healing

53. Write with Forefinger

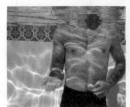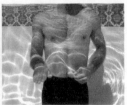

54. Hand Rotations

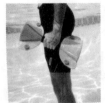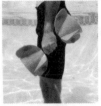

55. Lateral Hand Swings

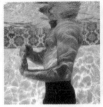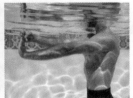

56. Wrist Flexor Stretch

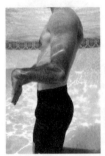

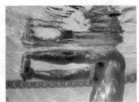

57. Wrist Extensor Stretch

58. Sponge Squeeze

The
Complete
Waterpower
Workout
Book

346

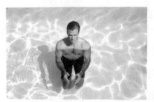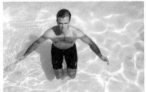

59. Arm Swings

See chart on pages 336 and 337 for numbers of sets and reps

Neck

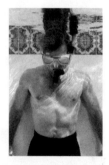

60. Submerged Neck Flexion and Extension

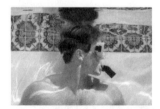

61. Submerged Rotations

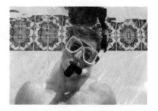

62. Submerged Neck Tilts

63. Submerged Partial Neck Circles

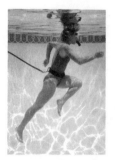

64. Submerged Water Running

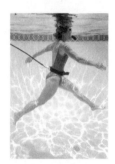

65. Submerged Water Walking

66. Submerged Intervals

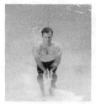 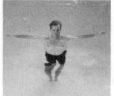

67. One-Way V Arm Lifts

Postsurgical
Water Healing

T w e l v e

The Return to Land

S ooner or later, you will return to your sport. During the long weeks or even months
of rehabilitation that follow serious injuries and surgeries, you may lose sight of
that. But the day *will* come, and you must plan for it and for the days to follow as
carefully as you planned your rehabilitation program.

During phases 1 and 2 of your rehabilitation, you work primarily in the pool. During
Phase 3, you begin introducing minimal amounts of land work. By the end of Phase 4,
you should be fully rehabilitated and ready for competition.

Determining when to begin Phase 3 may be your single most difficult decision if you
are supervising your own rehab. **Genuinely test the injury in the water before
trying your first land-based workout.** Push hard in the water by blasting a powerful
sprint in shallow water. Pump the arms and legs through the water with great strength
and speed. Jump high and swing the arms and legs in ways that you would be unsure
of on land. If you feel even a twinge of the former pain, don't return to land yet.

It is during Phase 3 that you must be extremely careful. Those first few days of
land-based activity, if overdone, could set you back to Phase 2 or even 1 again. So

The
Complete
Waterpower
Workout
Book

348

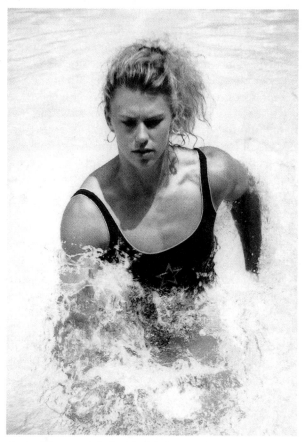

Genuinely test your injury before beginning land-based workouts.

continue your Water Healing Workouts and begin the limited land training as set forth in the suggested plan below.

Don't even consider returning to *full* land activities (Phase 4) until you have met these three critieria:

1. You have been performing Phase 3 activities pain free for at least two weeks.

2. You have regained 95 percent of your full strength in the injured area. Strength can be measured by single-leg or single-arm weight exercises. Compare your injured side to your healthy side. Do you feel muscle weakness in the "belly" (midpoint) of the muscle or at the attachment? Do you feel weakness in or around the joint? If so, you have not regained enough strength to return to land yet.

3. You have established 95 percent of your full flexibility in the injured body part. Again, compare the injured side to the healthy side to make your assessment. Look in the mirror as you reach, bend, and stretch. Do your arms reach equally high overhead? Can you see equal bend of the knees as you do a quad stretch? In a hamstring stretch, do your hands reach the same place on each leg?

If one side of your body is strong and flexible, it wants to perform up to capacity. If the other side is weak and stiff it can't keep up, but will try, which creates a potential for reinjury or fresh injury. So don't rush your comeback. If you begin full activity too soon, you risk entering the injury-reinjury cycle that becomes difficult to break. By giving yourself an extra week now, you may gain several months in the long run.

Memory can be your worst temptation during these crucial days and weeks. You *remember* how far you used to kick, how hard you used to hit, how fast you used to run. You will probably find that "used to" phrase in both your conversation and your thoughts. But as basketball legend Wilt Chamberlain always says, "Old man 'Used To' is dead and gone." What you *used to* do no longer applies. Forget it. Start with where you are.

Your first day back on land may be extremely short. In the case of a runner, it may be only four minutes long, then it's back to the pool for the rest of the workout. A football player might run slowly only one length of the field, then into the pool. A tennis player may hit with a partner for a mere five minutes the first day. Remember: You don't have to do your full workout on land anymore. You have learned how to satisfy your need for strenuous athletic output in the water and can always draw on that source if you need more activity than what your injury will allow you to do on land. You are continuing your Waterpower Workouts as you begin to re-create your "landability," sneaking up on your body with small pieces of your normal land activity. You can start with 5 percent land work and move up gradually, maintaining your physical and mental fitness by continuing concurrent high-powered Waterpower Workouts. This will best ensure that you avoid reinjury that is so common when athletes make a sudden jump back to activity.

It also ensures that you **avoid compensation injuries,** those problems that arise when the weakened or painful parts of your body force a shift of stresses to other body parts. For instance, when returning to land after an ankle sprain that has not been fully rehabilitated, an athlete may run with a limp. This altered gait places more stress on the lower back and the healthy leg, either of which can become strained. Or if a tennis player continues to play with a painful shoulder that alters his ground stroke, he will often develop elbow pain. So, don't resume your activity if you experience pain that alters your biomechanics. Concentrate on form to avoid compensation injuries.

Running is the universal conditioning activity and a major component of many sports. Athletes from virtually every sport use it as a primary method of increasing their fitness, so the plan set forth below uses running as the example. If you use a different basic conditioning activity, extrapolate from the example to suit your own needs.

Follow these basic guidelines:

- Don't re-create the injury by wearing the same shoes that may have contributed to the problem in the first place. Choose other, more trustworthy shoes. If you must buy new ones, break them in by wearing them around the house a few days before running in them.
- Go to a track or other smooth, flat surface. Don't try running on uneven terrain until you are well back into your routine. Avoid hills at all costs during this crucial transition.

The
Complete
Waterpower
Workout
Book

350

- Avoid overstriding. Too long a stride length keeps your body up in the air longer on each step, causing you to impact harder upon landing. Overstriding is not only inefficient, it can cause muscle or other soft-tissue strain. If you keep your running pace to approximately 180 steps per minute, you should avoid this pitfall.

- Protect the injured area. Heel lifts placed in running shoes take pressure off an Achilles tendon or calf injury and tape gives added support to a sprained ankle. As an everyday practice it's not advisable to rely on tape, a brace, or other appliances to prevent pain during a workout; however, they do provide a temporary measure of safety against reinjury during the first few land workouts.

- Wear a sports watch so you can time your workouts. Return-to-Land workouts use time rather than distance, which provides a built-in protection device. If you feel the need to run slowly on a given day, you may, for instance, cover only three quarters of a mile in eight minutes rather than a full mile. In this way, you don't try to go too far on a day when you are tired.

- If you cannot complete the suggested land-based workout on any given day, go immediately to the pool for a Deep Waterpower Workout to satisfy your craving for activity. Stay in deep water to eliminate further impact stress, and avoid any exercises that aggravate your injury.

- Work exceptionally hard on your water-training intervals. You want to quench your athletic thirst in the water so that you can be more relaxed about what you accomplish on land.

- Immediately before and after each land workout, perform a thorough stretch, concentrating on the injured area. Apply lavish amounts of ice to the area surrounding your former injury site. (See box, page 216.) Consider ice treatment any time you even suspect reaggravation of your injury or the beginning of a compensation injury.

- Follow the Hard/Easy Principle as set forth in Chapter 1. The program below adheres to that idea, providing enough rest time so your body can adapt to the new stresses.

- If you suspect that you ran too far or too fast and you might be sore tomorrow, go to the pool for a gentle Waterpower Warm-Down, which provides an extended-cool down and flushes out soreness. Ice the area immediately after the workout and again just before going to bed.

- Increase your land-training program *only* 10 to 20 percent in any given week.

- Run at a comfortable pace, whatever that may be. Don't add speed until it appears in Week 5.

- Return to Waterpower any day that land is scheduled if you feel a strain or suspect even minor reinjury. *Stay* in the water until that pain or strain is completely gone.

Week 1

Standard track coaching methodology calls for a short run before stretching so that the muscles are warmed up before they are asked to become pliable. But because of injuries, you will need to stretch before you do any activity on land. Injury sites need to be prepared for even the slightest work that is to follow.

For the first two weeks, days 1, 3, and 5 are your land workouts. If you can't complete the land workouts outlined below, do what you can. Days 2, 4, and 6 will be strictly water workouts. Day 7 is a rest day.

This plan is designed for those who train daily. If you work out only three times per week, do days 1, 2, and 3 in week 1, then continue alternating land and water workouts. Use the workouts suggested below for guidelines.

DAY 1

Stretch for at least five minutes. Walk fast for four minutes, then stretch the calves, hamstrings, and quads again. Spend extra time stretching your recovering injury site. Now try jogging slowly for one minute. Walk for one minute as you evaluate how you felt during this short run.

Did you experience pain or stiffness in the recovering injury area? Did you feel any other part of your body object to the run?

The
Complete
Waterpower
Workout
Book

352

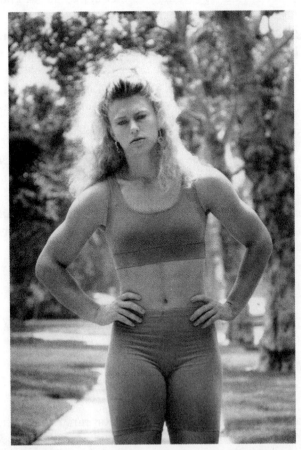

Carefully monitor your injury and return to the pool if you even suspect reinjury.

If the answer to either of those questions is yes, try to warm up those land-leery body parts with another one-minute jog. Walk another minute while you monitor your body and ask yourself these same questions. You may not get rid of the stiffness or slight pain this first day, but you may be able to work through at least eight one-minute runs before you feel you must discontinue. You will probably feel an awareness of or pressure in the former area of injury: That's normal. If the discomfort diminishes as you progress, good—it's warming up. If it hasn't lessened by the fourth one-minute interval, or if it becomes increasingly sore or painful, you'll have to make the decision to stop. If you feel pain, don't panic. All your disciplined rehab work wasn't wasted. You will probably tolerate your next run better. Remember that this is Day 1. Don't force a workout now that will cause a reinjury.

If you feel *any sharp pain,* terminate the workout. Return to water for a week before trying to return to land again. Perhaps you simply weren't ready yet. Be gentle with yourself. Remind yourself that you are doing all the right things: icing, stretching, and rehabilitating the area, and maintaining your fitness in the water. Don't panic!

If you answered no to the pain and stiffness questions above, you may be feeling surprisingly good after your first one-minute run. In that case, after walking a minute, try running two minutes, then walk a minute. Still feel good? Run another two minutes, then walk another minute. Run a maximum of four two-minute runs, then call it a day *no matter how good you feel.* **You won't know until later today or tomorrow how your body really tolerated the workout.**

DAY 2

Go back to the pool. If you felt any pain or stiffness during yesterday's workout, perform The Deep Waterpower Workout, Level 3, to avoid all weight bearing. Include in your interval section four strong one-minute runs and four fast one-minute walks. If you felt good on land, do The Waterpower Workout, Level 3, including in your interval section four strong two-minute runs. Recall the running mechanics you used yesterday and visualize yourself running on land.

DAY 3

Start again with a five-minute stretch, a four-minute fast walk, and another brief stretch. If you felt pain or stiffness on Day 1, try to work your way once again through a maximum of eight one-minute runs, walking one minute between. After two or three days of these runs, your body should start tolerating the movement and impact and start loosening up.

If you felt good on Day 1, begin with a preview one-minute run as before. If you still feel good, increase your run to four minutes, then walk two minutes. Run another four minutes, stretch and go home. If you still want to do more work, go to the pool. Don't start making grandiose plans for a 4-mile run yet. Do the disciplined work of following through on your Return-to-Land rehab plan so that you won't experience a flareup or reinjury.

DAY 4

Do The Deep Waterpower or Waterpower Workout, **Level 2.** Even though you may not think you need an easy day, your body is doing new things and needs a chance to adapt.

DAY 5

Repeat whatever you were able to accomplish on Day 3. Don't try to increase anything yet. Revel in the fact that *you are running.*

DAY 6

Choose either The Deep Waterpower Workout or The Waterpower Workout, Level 3, as you did on Day 2. Give yourself tough intervals that will tire you.

DAY 7

Rest. If you are compelled to do an active rest, perform The Deep or Shallow Waterpower Warm-Down and stretch.

You will probably fit in one of two possible "comeback" categories: (1) **Slow track:** those who must work slowly and gradually, and (2) **Fast track:** those who make rapid, easy gains in the first few weeks. You might not know which category you fit in until you've finished the first week and begun the second, so begin slowly. If the work still feels as hard on Day 1 of the second week, continue with the consistency of only a 10 to 20 percent increase each week until you experience a sudden breakthrough in function and feeling. But if you find that your running capability has returned and the injury feels as if it's behind you, increase your workout by 20 to 40 percent. Force yourself to listen to your body and adhere to your plan. By laying a disciplined base in the first few weeks, you increase your chances of making a smooth transition to land.

The
Complete
Waterpower
Workout
Book

354

Week 2

DAY 1

Slow track. Those who are still somewhat stiff and sore can try adding 10 to 20 percent to the workout. If you were running eight one-minute runs, increase to nine, maintaining a one-minute walk between intervals.

Fast track. Those who feel quick improvement can add 20 to 40 percent. Try running three four-minute runs. Walk two minutes between runs. Even if you still feel good, call it a day.

DAY 2

Slow track. The Deep Waterpower Workout, Level 3. Intervals: three-minute buildup run (increase speed each minute) and three-minute buildup walk (increase speed each minute).

Fast track. The Waterpower Workout, Level 3. Intervals: five *fast* one-minute runs.

DAY 3

Slow track. Same as Day 1.

Fast track. Two six-minute runs (three-minute walk between) on Day 3. You'll probably be tempted to start picking up the pace. Don't. Not yet.

DAYS 4 AND 6

The Deep Waterpower or Waterpower Workout. Same as Day 2, but vary the intervals to stay mentally fresh.

DAY 5

Slow track. Increase to four two-minute runs.

Fast Track. Two seven-minute runs at the same gentle pace (three-minute walk between).

DAY 7

Rest or stretch.

In the middle of a workout, somewhere around the third or fourth week, you're going to have the thought: "I can run six miles again—today!" **Don't.** If you retain your caution and deliberateness throughout this Return-to-Land period, your progress will generally be steady and consistent. An occasional setback—pain, undue soreness—may require an unprogrammed day or two in the pool. Don't get upset; just do the work. It's all part of the normal comeback.

If you are rehabbing from a serious injury or surgery, you have probably already sensed that the alternating land and water workouts are serving you well. In that case, repeat weeks 1 and 2 before increasing your land days as in Week 3 below. Don't rush the comeback. You *are* getting your workouts in the pool.

Week 3

From the third to the fourth week, never do more than two consecutive days on land. (Land, Land, Water, Land, Land, Water, Rest)

DAYS 1 AND 2

Slow track. If you are still working through stiffness and soreness, continue with the same work load as Week 2: four two-minute runs with two-minute walks between.

Fast track. If you feel good and are ready to increase your work load, add 20 to 40 percent: a seven-minute run, a three-minute walk, a six-minute run, a three-minute walk, and a five-minute run. Walk two to three minutes between each of these runs.

DAY 3

The Deep Waterpower Workout, Level 2, for everyone. Eliminate all impact after two straight days of land work.

DAYS 4 AND 5

Slow track. Add 10 to 20 percent so that now you run three three-minute runs with a two-minute walk between.

Fast track. Comfortably run seven minutes, walk three minutes, run seven minutes, walk three minutes, and run four minutes. The total running time adds up to eighteen minutes. You can vary the segments as long as you keep them in three pieces, broken by three-minute walks. If you crave more, satisfy that appetite in the pool. Don't add speed yet. You're still building your mobility base. Think: **Slow, but sure.**

DAY 6

If you feel like more work, choose The Waterpower Workout, Level 2. If you're fatigued, choose The Waterpower Warm-Down.

The
Complete
Waterpower
Workout
Book

356

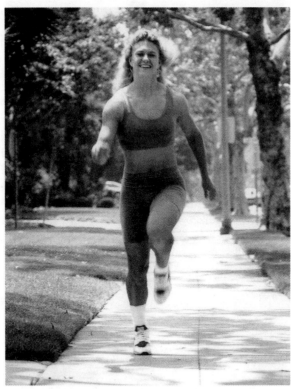

There will be a day you will feel great again, successfully making your return to land.

DAY 7

Rest or stretch.

Week 4

Continue with the same plan as in Week 3. The work load remains constant this week, but if you are feeling good, you can carefully begin to increase your speed. Don't try sprinting or even powerfully striding yet. Midway through a workout, select one of your running intervals and step up your pace by only *one* gear. In the next workout you may try for *one* faster gear. Never jump up two or three gears at a time. **Step up one gear at a time.** If you are accustomed to clocking your workouts, don't try to measure up to performances you could achieve prior to your injury. Let your body, not your stopwatch, dictate the speed of each run.

Weeks 5 through 8

If yours was a serious injury or if you had surgery, you will want to repeat the program set forth in weeks 3 and 4: Land, Land, Water, Land, Land, Water. This allows your body gradually to become accustomed to the demands of working once again against gravity. Then, if you're doing well with the program outlined above, continue to increase your work load 5 to 10 percent a week as long as you are injury free.

Once you return to your full preinjury routine, retain at least one weekly Waterpower Workout Session, preferably midweek in your program to break up the daily pounding on your weight-bearing joints. Perform a Waterpower Warm-Down after every high-intensity land workout, and prudently prescribe Waterpower for yourself whenever you suspect the possibility of strain or injury. Practice your sport-specific drills in water and follow the hard/easy and periodization principles set forth in Chapter 1.

By learning to use water wisely in your fitness routine, you will cut down the severity of training injuries. You will speed your recovery back to your land activities, and you will always be glad you made such a dependable friend in water.

**The
Complete
Waterpower
Workout
Book**

358

Appendix

The following is a list of manufacturers and their products, which appeared in the text:

1. Aqua Energetics
500 N. Union Street
Middletown, PA 17057
(717) 944-5515
Fax: (717) 657-1566

PRODUCT: HydroWorx hydro therapy tank
Small tank for clinic or home use

2. Aqua Source
6112 N. Covington
Oklahoma City, OK 73132
(405) 722-2651
Fax: (405) 722-4884

PRODUCT: Aqua Belt
Flotation belt for deep-water exercise

3. Aqua Therapeutics, Inc.
P.O. Box 5775
Asheville, NC 28813
(704) 252-8268 & (704) 377-9109
Fax: (704) 332-3044

PRODUCT: Aquatoner
Adjustable resistance equipment
to be hand held or strapped to a
leg

4. Aqua Tunes
1020 Berea Drive
Boulder, CO 80303
(303) 494-7224

PRODUCT: Aqua Tunes
Waterproof case for cassette
player

5. Aquarius Health & Fitness Products, Inc.

Plaza 222 South U.S. Highway
One
Suite 202
Tequesta, FL 33469
(407) 743-6550
Fax: (407) 743-6554

PRODUCTS: Aquarius water workout
station
A multi-use, in-pool, stainless steel
exercise station
Aquarius water workout tank
Small tank for clinic or home use

6. Bodyciser International Corporation

511 River Drive
Elmwood Park, NJ 07407
(201) 791-9601
Fax: (201) 791-0452

PRODUCTS: Bodyciser
A therapeutic flotation mattress
Hol-Tite restrainer
A portable handle to stick on
pool walls

7. Bioenergetics

2841 Anode Lane
Dallas, TX 75220
(214) 350-1333
Fax: (214) 352-9449

PRODUCTS: Wet Vest, Wet Vest II,
Wet Belt
Flotation vests and belt for
deep-water exercise

8. D.K. Douglas Company, Inc.

299 Bliss Road
Longmeadow, MA 01106
(413) 567-8572
Fax: (413) 567-3153

PRODUCT: Wet Wrap
A vest for warmth

9. Excel Sports Science

P.O. Box 5612
Eugene, OR 97405
(800) 922-9544
(503) 484-2454
Fax: (503) 484-0501

PRODUCT: Aqua Jogger
A flotation belt for deep-water
exercise with special design for
lower back support

10. Hydro-Fit, Inc.

440 Charnelton
Eugene, OR 97401
(503) 484-4361 & (800) 346-7295
Fax: (503) 484-1443

PRODUCTS: Hydro-Fit Buoyancy
Cuffs and Hand Buoys
Flotation devices that fit on ankles
and are hand-held

11. Hydro-Tone Intl, Inc.

6125 W. Reno
Suite 900
Oklahoma City, OK 73127
(405) 789-7717 & (800) 622-8663
Fax: (405) 789-7795

PRODUCTS: Hydro-Tone boots and
bells
High-resistance equipment that is
hand-held and put on feet for
upper and lower body exercises

12. J&B Foam Fabricators, Inc.

111 So. Jebavy Drive, PO Box 144
Ludington, MI 49431
(616) 843-2448 & (800) 621-3626
Fax: (616) 843-8723

PRODUCTS: Instructional Swim Bar,
Water Wafer, Kick Board, Foam pieces
that provide flotation and resistance

13. Nuvo Sport, Inc.

4954 Sauquoit Lane
Annandale, VA 22003
(703) 914-0637
Fax: (703) 914-0370

The
Complete
Waterpower
Workout
Book

360

PRODUCT: SpaBells
Versatile hand-held devices that
can be used for flotation or
adjustable resistance

14. NZ Mfg., Inc.
7405 S. 212th St., Unit 125
Kent, WA 98032
(800) 886-6621

PRODUCT: StrechCordz
Stretchable tethers of all lengths
for in-place swimming
Waterpower Workout Tether
Designed by Lynda Huey for in-place
water running and walking
Order from Huey's Athletic Network
(310) 829-5622
Fax: (310) 828-5401

15. One Stop Brace Shop
(310) 824-6464

PRODUCT: Stealth custom knee
brace
Waterproof, anatomically hinged
rigid brace for all sports and
water therapy

16. Polar CIC Inc.
99 Seaview Blvd.
Port Washington, NY 11050
(516) 484-2400
Fax: (516) 484-2789

PRODUCTS: Accurex and Edge heart
monitors
Water-proof chest strap and wrist
watch to monitor heart rate

17. Sports Fit International
7755 Fay Avenue
Suite C
La Jolla, CA 92037
(619) 459-3221
Fax: (619) 459-8588

PRODUCT: ICE 'N' HEAT
Freezeable and microwaveable gel
pack plus fabric wrap with velcro
straps

18. Speedo America
7911 Haskell Ave.
Van Nuys, CA 91409
(800) 547-8770
Fax: (818) 373-4274
Fax: (818) 373-4433

PRODUCT: Speedo SwimMitt XT
Cross-Training Gloves
Neoprene webbed glove with
compartments to add weights,
which offers resistance below and
above water

19. SwimEx Systems
P.O. Box 328
Warren, RI 02885
(401) 245-7946
Fax: (401) 245-3160

PRODUCT: SwimEx Hydrotherapy
Pools
Small tank for clinic or home use

20. Tabaka Aqua Golf
Order from Huey's Athletic
Network
(310) 829-5622
Fax: (310) 828-5401

PRODUCT: Swing Trainer
Water golf club for practicing golf
swing

21. Texas Recreation Corporation
P.O. Box 539
Wichita Falls, TX 76307
(800) 433-0956
Fax: (817) 723-8505

PRODUCT: Wet Sweat Belt
Teal-colored flotation belt for
deep-water exercise

Index

About the Authors

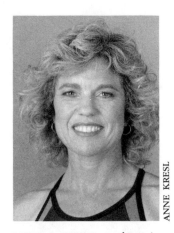

ANNE KRESL

LYNDA HUEY was born in Vallejo, California. She was educated at San Jose State University, where she was the school's outstanding female sprinter and trained with the famed "Speed City" group of male Olympic sprinters. She taught and coached at California Polytechnic State University, Oberlin College, Los Angeles City College, Santa Monica College, and UCLA. Her autobiography *A Running Start: An Athlete, a Woman* was published in 1976. For nearly ten years Lynda wrote for many sports magazines, hosted her own sports radio show on Santa Monica's National Public Radio station KCRW, and in 1988 she worked for NBC at the Seoul Olympic Games. Her own athletic injuries led her to water rehabilitation and in 1986 she published *The Waterpower Workout*. That same year she opened Huey's Athletic Network, a coaching and consulting business in Santa Monica specializing in water training programs for fitness, cross training, and healing. Lynda consults with hospitals, schools, and health clubs in designing swimming pools, establishing therapy programs, and training personnel. She is a world-renowned lecturer and leader in the water-fitness industry, and in 1992 received an award from the United States Water Fitness Association created in her name. Each year the Lynda Huey Award will be given to a leader in the field of athletic water rehabilitation. Some of the athletes and entertainers Lynda has helped rehabilitate include: Florence Griffith Joyner, Wilt Chamberlain, Bo Jackson, Mike Powell, John Lloyd, Valerie Brisco, Paula Abdul, Kathy Smith, Cybill Shepherd, Sinbad, and Juliet Prowse.

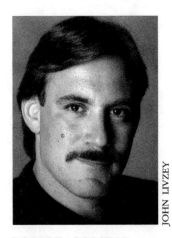

JOHN LIVZEY

ROBERT FORSTER was raised in Pearl River, New York. He began his education in the health sciences at Bloomsberg State College in Pennsylvania where he also competed on the school's prominent N.C.A.A. Division I wrestling team. In 1980 he graduated with honors from the Physical Therapy Program of the State University of New York at Stony Brook.

Upon graduation he moved to Los Angeles, where he worked with the nation's leading sports medicine hospitals and doctors before opening a private practice in Santa Monica. Since the 1984 Olympics his clinic has served as a training and treatment center for Olympic athletes from all over the world.

At the last three Olympics he has served as the personal physical therapist providing on site "event coverage" for Coach Bob Kersee and his athletes, including Jackie Joyner-Kersee, Valerie Brisco, Florence "Flo-Jo" Griffith Joyner, Jeanette Bolden, Greg Foster, Andre Phillips, Al Joyner, and Gail Devers. Together these athletes have won twenty-three Olympic medals.

Robert has lectured extensively on sports and dance physical therapy and rehabilitation throughout the United States and Europe and serves on the board of advisors for *Fitness Magazine*. He has made significant contributions to the safety aspects of aerobic exercise and fitness programs while serving as a consultant on book and video projects by such leaders in the fitness industry as Gilda Marx and Kathy Smith.

About the Photographer

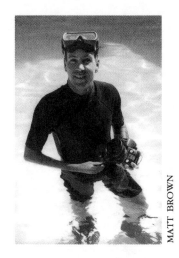

MATT BROWN

PHOTOGRAPHER PETE ROMANO is owner of Hydro-Flex in Los Angeles, a research and development facility specializing in professional underwater motion picture cameras and lighting equipment for the rental market. Pete began his career as an underwater cameraman in the United States Navy. Since 1979 he has worked in Hollywood on feature films, TV shows, and commercials, shooting the underwater segments in such movies as *Splash, Star Trek IV, The Abyss, Always, Cape Fear, Point Break, Prince of Tides, Dracula,* and *Free Willy.* Pete Romano recommended Lynda Huey to Barbra Streisand as someone who could train the children actors for their underwater sequence in her movie *Prince of Tides.*

In the past year, Pete has suffered two very serious breaks in his left femur. Each time, he entered the water for daily Water

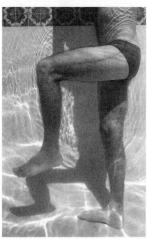

LYNDA HUEY

Healing Workouts with Lynda Huey and amazed the surgeons with his rapid recovery of strength, flexibility, and full function. Pete Romano has *lived* the importance of this book.

About the Type

This book was set in Garamond, a typeface designed by the French printer Jean Jannon. It is styled after Garamond's original models. The face is dignified, and is light but without fragile lines. The italic is modeled after a font of Granjon, which was probably cut in the middle of the sixteenth century.